Mediter
Di

2 Manuscripts

Mediterranean diet for beginners + Alkaline diet

The complete guide for weight loss, burn fats and live healthy

<u>Simone Press</u>

By reading this document, the reader agrees that under no circumstances is the author responsible for any losses, direct or indirect, which are incurred as a result of the use of information contained within this document, including, but not limited to, — errors, omissions, or inaccuracies.

Mediterranean Diet for Beginners

- The Complete Guide -

The Diet Plan for Weight Loss. Delicious Recipes for Living and Eating Healthy

\+

Alkaline Diet

The Complete Guide for Beginners. Eat well with Alkaline Diet Cookbook.

Delicious Alkaline Recipes

Table of Contents

BOOK 1: MEDITERRANEAN DIET FOR BEGINNERS

BOOK 2. ALKALINE DIET

Book 1
Mediterranean Diet for Beginners

- The Complete Guide -

The Diet Plan for Weight Loss. Delicious Recipes for Living and Eating Healthy

Introduction

When you hear the words, Mediterranean diet, what images come to mind? You will likely think of olive oil on everything, beautiful blue waters, stucco buildings, and sunny beaches. Maybe you have gotten to witness the beauty of the countries surrounding the Mediterranean Sea.

Have you ever wished there was a diet that didn't come with a strict menu that made you starve yourself? Could you believe that there is one, which provides you with delicious and diverse foods? The Mediterranean diet can provide you with all of this. The Mediterranean diet is said to be the healthiest diet on earth. It is full of nutritious foods, more so than any of those other diets that come with a list of foods you can't eat. With the Mediterranean diet, you get to enjoy grains, vegetables, and fruits. You can also enjoy fats, spices and herbs, poultry, fish, and meats in moderation. You can even enjoy a glass of wine if you so choose to. Add in some regular physical activity, and you have a recipe for a healthy lifestyle and weight loss.

The Mediterranean diet comes from the eating habits of the countries that surround the Mediterranean Sea, mostly coming from Spain, France, Greece, and Southern Italy. That means it is not only a diet but traditions. It has been proven to help with weight loss, lower the risk of dementia and depress, and prevent heart attacks. This is a lifestyle that everybody can benefit from.

It is important that you learn everything about a diet before you start to follow it. This book will provide you with the information that you need concerning the Mediterranean diet, how it came to be, the main foods you can eat, and some other important information that can help you.

Not only will you learn everything you need to about the Mediterranean diet, but you will also find a lot of delicious recipes that you can start enjoying right away. The recipes are simple, easy, and delicious. The best thing is that most of them won't take all that long to cook.

More likely than not, once you make it through this book, you will start to fill your plate up with delicious, colorful foods that are based on the Mediterranean principles.

There are plenty of books on this subject on the market, so thanks again for choosing this one! Every effort was made to ensure it is full of as much useful information as possible. Please enjoy!

Mediterranean Diet

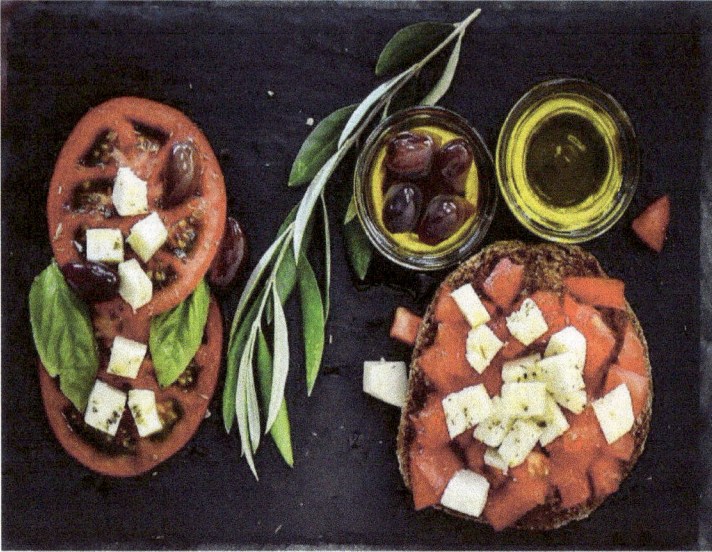

Whenever anyone hears "diet" imagines a strict list of foods that they aren't allowed to eat. When anybody hears "the Mediterranean diet" they imagine a sea, fresh air, exotic fruits, and unending beaches. This image can be inspiring and helps you begin to understand the Mediterranean diet.

Most people know that the people who live in the countries that border the Mediterranean Sea do live a lot longer and don't suffer from cardiovascular problems and cancer. Their secret is a diet that is low in saturated fat, sugar, and red meat, weight control, and active lifestyles. Their diets are loaded with nuts, produce, and healthy foods. This diet offers many benefits like diabetes control and prevention, cancer prevention, brain and heart health, and weight loss. If you follow the Mediterranean diet, you can keep weight off and stay away from chronic diseases.

The Mediterranean diet isn't a typical diet; it is the lifestyle habits and nutrition of the cultures that live near the Mediterranean Sea. There isn't just one Mediterranean diet, either. The Italians eat different foods than the Greeks; these eat different foods than the Spanish and French. They all share most of the same principles. Many people believe the Mediterranean diet isn't a diet but a habit to be learned over one's lifetime. France, Spain, Greece, and Italy all have cuisines that are unique to them, but they all share some common principles such as fresh foods during each season. These foods are very healthy and useful.

Cost of this Diet

How much the Mediterranean diet costs is just like any other aspect of life, it all depends on the way you shape it. Some ingredients like fresh produce, fish, nuts, and olive oil can get expensive, but there are ways to keep the cost down. Since you will be replacing red meats with more plant-based cooking and cooking more from home, you will be saving money there. Your choices when shopping will matter, too. If you can't afford a $50 red wine, grab one you can afford. Purchase your vegetables when they are on sale instead of paying full price.

How it Works

Everybody knows how important a balanced diet is to keep us healthy. Due to our crazy lives, not many people can follow a healthy diet. They find quick and easy foods when it comes to making meals.

This isn't a structured diet but an eating pattern. You have to figure out the number of calories you need to eat in order to lose weight or maintain your weight. You have to decide what you need to do for exercise and the way you will make your own menu.

This diet emphasizes eating olive oil, legumes, nuts, beans, whole grains, vegetables, fruits along with flavorful spices and herbs. Seafood and fish are eaten a few times each week. You will eat yogurt, cheese, eggs, and poultry in moderation. Red meats and sweets are saved for special occasions. Top all this off with some red wine and exercise, and you have a foundation for success.

The red wine isn't a necessity but having one glass each day for women or two for men is great as long as your doctor says so. Red wine is great for us because it has resveratrol in it. This is a compound that can add years to your life. You would have to drink a huge amount to get enough to make any difference. This diet doesn't involve any difficult or extraordinary foods, and you won't even have to take any supplements. This diet emphasizes seafood, nuts, whole grains vegetables, and fruits. It replaces bad fats with olive oil. It contrasts to other diets because it doesn't limit any foods or products. It encourages you to eat various foods in moderation. It is very important to eat high-quality foods in small amounts. These foods are very nourishing but keep you from eating too much. By doing this, the Mediterranean diet is great for people who struggle with weight problems. You can reach weight loss goals while enjoying delicious foods.

Here are a few general rules about the Mediterranean diet:

- Exercise more

- Eat about four eggs every week

- Consume no more than two glasses of red wine daily

- Eat nuts for a snack

- Consume pork and red meat a few times every month

- Consume nut butter instead of dairy butter

- Yogurts, cheese, and milk need to be low fat

- Eat shellfish and fish four or more times a week

- Get rid of white flour and use whole grain flour

- Instead of using margarine and butter use extra virgin olive oil

- Eat more seasonal vegetables and fruits

The Mediterranean diet is one of the healthiest diets around. This diet is great to follow even if you think that switching to low-fat dairy and fish and staying away from fast food is going to be hard. Some diet plans won't meet your expectations in spite of all their big words and promises. But rest easy, this diet will change your life if you can only make an effort. It will make you happy and healthy.

Exercise

Exercise is required when following the Mediterranean diet, but you don't have to make it feel like an exercise. Walking is a great place to begin. You can add whatever you like to do into your day. It might be Pilates, yoga, running, swimming, boxing, whatever, and you do what you like to do. Choose something you can stick with. Adults need to do a few days of weight lifting each week along with some moderate intensity exercises.

Origins

On the island of Pantelleria, time stands still. This island is located along the Mediterranean Sea. It is 65 miles from Sicily's coast and 36 miles away from North Africa. There aren't any taxis that travel around this little island since it is just six miles wide and nine miles long. It is made of black volcanic rock that came from ancient volcanoes and sits against the sea's waters that run green. Many black rock terraces run along slopes that look like tiers of a wedding cake. Low black stone cottages with vaulted white domes create spots on a hill. There are only about 8,000 locals. They are vibrant and warm and possess a relaxed and slow nature that most people possess in this piece of the world.

Not many tourists have found this "black pearl" even though it is a hideaway for architects and designers. Pantelleria's best feature is its cuisine that focuses on regionally sourced foods like spices, herbs, capers, and olives. They lean heavily on traditions that have been passed down from generation to generation. This is the foundation of this diet.

Many people consider the diets of the people that surround the Mediterranean Sea to be a "poor man's diet." It has been developed over centuries while people labor to make food from the inhospitable terrain. During the prehistoric times, inhabitants raised and hunted animals. During the Bronze Age, they began clearing the land for farming. This has been their primary source of food through history to this day. About one thousand years ago, the people began stacking up lava rocks to form a perfectly constructed wall that curves around the island. Each slope on each hill was terraced to protect and contain the soil from erosion. It also helps to capture each drop of moisture. The terraces make an ecosystem that is unique where caper plants and grapevines flourish. These terraces still serve as a great tool for farming plus offer a charming feature to their land.

Another architectural and agricultural feature on the island is the Giardino Pantesco. This is a dry enclosure that is made of stone. It can be oval, square, or round and it creates an ideal climate that is needed to grow citrus fruits. This dates back to when the Arab's dominated the island. There are about 1,500 of these "secret" gardens that still stand on Pantelleria. These treasures create a rustic charm, but their value comes from the quest for survival by shaping the environment that will sustain the human body. The people from this small island had to face constant winds, very little rainfall, and rocky terrain. The enclosed gardens and terraces made a buffer for the wind while collecting moisture from dew to give the ground hydration without the need for irrigation. The enclosed gardens and terraces show the determination and ingenuity that these people were made to create their regional diet.

All the plants grow horizontally and low to the ground. They are very well protected from the wind. At the roots of every grapevine, you will find a basin that collects the dew that goes to the roots. This technique was created hundreds of years ago. One treasured plant is the caper. It can sprout like a weed in a crack of a rock that hangs over the sea or an unlikely place. These capers have very intense flavors and are preserved and fermented in sea salt and not vinegar.

Another treasured plant is the olive tree. This is the symbol that unites the three religions in this region: Islam, Judaism, and Christianity. Olive trees only grow to a height of two feet tall. They grow out instead of up.

If it couldn't be grown, they didn't eat it. This is true for most of the foods in this diet. Harsh climates limited the number of crops that gets produced but in turn, gives them intense flavors. There has always been a great inventiveness and creativity to this diet. Wild herbs, potatoes, peppers, zucchinis, and tomatoes are just a few of the vegetables that grow here. Staples like chickpeas, lentils, barley, and wheat also grow here. Many people will grow almonds in their gardens at home.

Local diets along the Mediterranean have been shaped by various cultures from Italian to Arabian. This region has been the crossroad for many cultures and civilizations. These islands were created by volcanoes 250,000 years ago. The very first settlers came from North Africa in 3,000 B.C. The Romans occupied this region during the third century BC, and it was visited by the Carthaginians and Phoenicians.

Pirates plundered the island for hundreds of years. Muslim farmers settled it around 860 AD and planted citrus trees and grapes. The Arabs were exiled in 1090, and it has changed hands many times during the next few hundred years. French cuisine was introduced to Sicily during the Napoleonic wars and was married with the local foods. Traditional dishes mirror the many cultural influences and the availability of food.

History

The name for this diet comes from two words that we will take a closer look at so we will be able to understand this diet better.

Mediterranean: this is the sea's name that sits between Africa, Asia, and Europe. It only has one natural entry from the west at the Atlantic Ocean and a manmade exit at the east toward the Red Sea. This sea's name was given to it from the Latins. During the third century, Solinos named the sea "Mare Mediterraneum." This means "sea in between two continents." This became the name of the sea because in Latin "Mare" means sea.

In the countries that surround the Mediterranean Sea, we see how the Mediterranean diet was established. Olive trees grow in abundance here, and fruits are in season year-round because of the mild climate. Fish was a part of their diet, and many people were fishermen by trade. The herbs that grew there weren't just used to cook with but had medicinal purposes, too that saved people's lives.

Many ancient civilizations flourished here, and great empires such as the Roman Empire originated here.

Diet: The way we commit to the Mediterranean diet can get stronger if we understand the word "diet." The word "diet" usually carries negativity with it because people hear the word diet and automatically think limited food supply. This isn't the case with the Mediterranean diet. The origin of "diet" comes from the Greek word "diaita" that means a way of living or way of life.

Basically, this is saying the ancient Greek word "diaita" meaning "way of living" wasn't referring to or restricting the dietary habits or needs of their people. It was referring to the entire spectrum of life: activities, social environment, companions, sleep, work, and where you live.

When people follow the Mediterranean diet, it means they have agreed to follow a healthy living plant that might not cause weight loss, but it will dictate a way to live that puts them on the right track for healthy outcomes.

The Mediterranean diet has existed for hundreds of years, and many could argue that it's the oldest diet out there because it has been alive for over three thousand years. The basics of this diet come from the daily diets of the people who live in Cyprus, Spain, Portugal, Greece, France, and Italy. This diet incorporates cultural varieties while creating a rich lifestyle. The Mediterranean diet is the best eating routine in the world. This diet's main elements were created over hundreds of years. Many of the people in this region were farmers who cultivated olives and grapes. Some people were fishermen. People in this region didn't eat dairy or beef due to the bad climate conditions for these animals.

This isn't some new-fangled diet, and maybe that is why it is so widespread and popular. After numerous centuries, the way these people eat hasn't changed and has kept all the main elements.

Dr. Ancel Keys was the scientist who studied this diet, in 1958. He started looking at heart-healthy lifestyles and diets. He researched mortality rates and diseases in seven nations over a span of fifteen years.

His results showed the death rate in the Mediterranean region was a lot lower when compared to the United States. He realized the reason behind this their eating habits and lifestyle.

Many other studies have shown the same effects when following the Mediterranean diet. They also confirmed this diet could lower a person's type 2 diabetes, heart problems, and obesity levels.

The Mediterranean Life

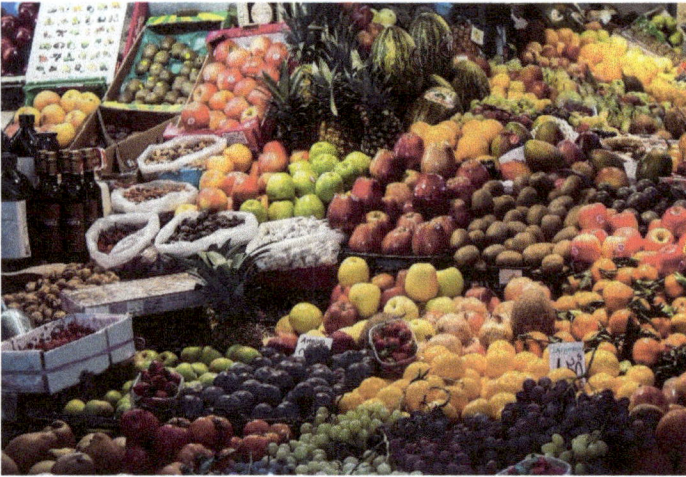

The Mediterranean diet does have some anti-inflammatory properties, low-fat products, and foods that are plant-based. Getting exercise and not smoking are necessary in order to achieve prosperity.

It is heavy with vegetables and fruit, but this diet allows you to be happy, drink, and eat. There are some advantages to following this diet:

- Lessens heart problems

This diet has been proven to help with symptoms of heart problems and other chronic illnesses. It decreases the mortality rate due to cardiovascular failure since it lowers bad cholesterol. These are the low-density lipoprotein that carries the fat molecules through the body in extracellular water. The benefits are more obvious with people in higher socioeconomic statuses. If your Mediterranean lifestyle stays away from saturated fat and includes healthy poly-and monounsaturated fats moderately, you are doing your heart a huge favor. The huge impact on heart health is because of the use of olive oil. People who consume extra virgin olive oil will have lower blood pressure than people who consume sunflower oil.

Red wine, when drunk moderately, can also reduce heart disease.

Dr. Ancel Keys began learning about the benefits of the Mediterranean diet during the 1950s but didn't become popular until the 1990s. He realized that people who lived in the poor region of southern Italy had lower risks of death due to heart disease than wealthy people who lived in New York. He attributed this to what they ate.

Other factors like being more active could have impacted this along with the reduction of sugars, and red meat have been linked to lower chances of coronary heart disease and stroke. This is due to the monounsaturated fats that are found in the Mediterranean lifestyle with all the vegetables and fruits that are consumed.

Monounsaturated fats help the function and concentration of good cholesterol in the blood. This balances cholesterol and helps to defend the heart.

- Helps type 2 diabetes

This lifestyle is a great option to help prevent and control diabetes. Being overweight is a huge factor in type 2 diabetes. If you want to lose weight and be able to keep it off, the Mediterranean lifestyle can help you do that. You will certainly tilt the scales in your favor. Following a healthy Mediterranean lifestyle could reduce or reverse any risk of developing a metabolic syndrome that leads to heart disease and type 2 diabetes. When it is compared to high protein, vegan, and vegetarian diets, the Mediterranean diet is great for people who have high blood sugar or diabetes. Olive oil and plant-based foods help to decrease cholesterol and blood sugar. The Mediterranean diet doesn't have a lot of sugar in it since the only sugar you consume comes in the form of an occasional dessert, wine, and fruit.

Studies have been done on the risks of developing specific diseases according to what they eat. People who followed the Mediterranean diet was compared to others who eat the Northern European or American diet.

Results showed the Mediterranean habits help to keep certain genetic mutations that might lead to having a stroke, especially if someone carries two copies of a specific gene. Olive oil and wine showed antioxidant properties that protected against hardening of the blood vessels or atherosclerosis. More research is being done to confirm this benefit.

A study done by Italian scientists linked the fiber and antioxidants in this diet with good physical and mental health.

Lifestyle

The Mediterranean lifestyle is very nutritious. A buffet of Mediterranean foods will include healthy foods such as olive oil, salmon, vegetables, fruits, salads, hummus, and pita. This lifestyle meets the US government's nutrition recommendations. Research has found that this lifestyle can help preserve your brain's volume as you age.

The federal government recommends that women consume around 2,200 calories per day while men need to consume 2, 600. The Mediterranean diet recommends your daily intake of calories is around 1,500 whether you are a woman or man. Since this diet is very individualized, your intake is going to vary.

Here are five basics to live the Mediterranean lifestyle:

1. Following the diet

Following the Mediterranean diet is as easy as grabbing a handful of nuts, having fresh vegetables, or a bowl of lentil soup for a snack. Twice a week, try to eat seafood or fish for dinner with a side of grains or rice with a chopped salad to begin the meal. You can have lean cuts of meat like poultry in moderation and red meats occasionally. There are occasional pastries, cakes, and chocolate. What's a meal without baklava? Having dried or fresh fruit is seen more frequently as a choice for dessert.

With all the varieties that the pyramid allows, it is hard to think about this way of eating as a diet. There aren't any food restrictions with this lifestyle. Most foods are allowed. On their pyramid, you will see that vegetables and grains are eaten the most, and then comes dairy. You will get lean proteins and fiber from seafood and nuts. Olive oil is the main source of fat, and a little wine is always allowed.

2. Be with people you love

Share with people you love. Spend time with family. When talking about eating on the Mediterranean diet, it is all about portion size. A good habit is not eating alone. Eat your meals at a table surrounded by friends and family. When you share meals with others, you will eat slower, and you won't stuff yourself.

Beyond sharing meals, it also encourages having a balanced social life and being connected to people who matter to you. You might go out with friends and socialize with a lot of people. This isn't the kind of life the Mediterranean diet talks about. You need to surround yourself with family and a few friends who mean the most to you. These people need to be loyal to you. They need to care deeply for you. They are the ones who tell you the truth and help you grow. This frees up your social calendar, but your social life becomes a lot richer.

3. Naturally, move

Most Mediterranean people don't actually exercise. They don't take two hours out of their day to lift weights or go to the gym. This doesn't mean they are inactive.

In that part of the world, not many things are convenient, so moving is natural for people who live there. They do manual labor, they climb upstairs, they walk, and I mean a lot. They will walk to work. They walk to the dairy shop, bakery, or market. They walk to friend's houses. They go for a walk if they are looking for something leisurely to do. Many people do not even own cars.

If you have a gym membership, please don't stop going. Most of the people who join a gym will quit within a month. Utilizing natural movement, doing moderate exercise like going for a daily walk is very effective and can become a healthy habit. If you do yoga now, please continue just try to walk a bit more.

4. Laugh more

Most people have heard the old saying "laughter is the best medicine." This is so very true with the Mediterranean lifestyle. It isn't the main character of every person who lives in the Mediterranean region, but it is evident in many. These people have huge personalities. They love telling stories, and these conversations are filled with lots of humor. You can take life seriously but do it with joy.

5. Live Simply

Many of the people who live in France, Turkey, Greece, and Egypt don't have that many possessions. They make conservative decisions about their daily needs. They never buy too much of any one ingredient. The thought of buying anything in bulk is completely foreign to them. Eating what is fresh is what matters. They don't fret over making more than one trip to the market. They will do it on foot, too. Recipes such as paella where they turn leftovers into a flavor-packed dish and fattoush that is made from day-old bread are examples of ways to minimize waste and create tasty meals.

The Mediterranean Diet Pyramid

You can find the guidelines for the Mediterranean diet in the "Mediterranean Diet Pyramid." It is the standard dietary plan that can boost your health.

This pyramid was made in 1993 and is what gave this diet its popularity. It was created by Oldways Preservation and Exchange Trust and the Harvard School of Public Health. Oldways is an organization that specializes in promoting healthy nutrition.

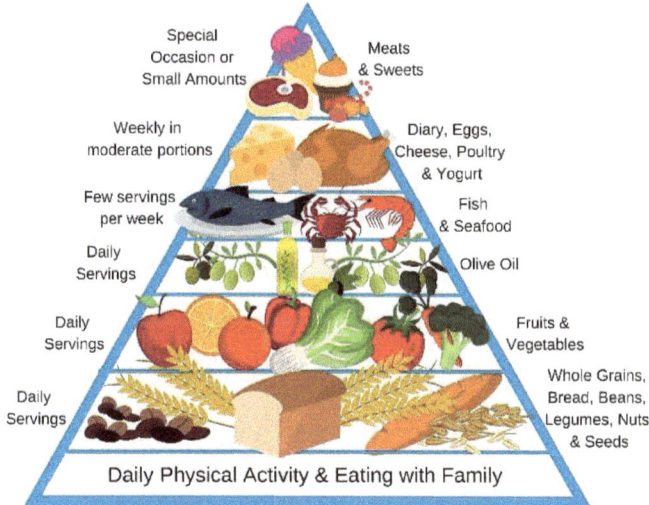

Special Occasion or Small Amounts — Meats & Sweets

Weekly in moderate portions — Diary, Eggs, Cheese, Poultry & Yogurt

Few servings per week — Fish & Seafood

Daily Servings — Olive Oil

Daily Servings — Fruits & Vegetables

Daily Servings — Whole Grains, Bread, Beans, Legumes, Nuts & Seeds

Daily Physical Activity & Eating with Family

MEDITERRANEAN DIET

This pyramid reflects the cultural and social traditions of the Mediterranean region. It is a lot more than placing foods in order due to its importance. It explores ways to serve, cook, and choosing foods. The quality of food and portion sized need attention, too.

The pyramid's base shows how important it is to have strong social connections, sharing meals with friends and family, and exercise. You need to put exercise as a priority especially exercises like aerobics and running. Small activities like walking upstairs, housework, and walking the dog can contribute a lot to your health.

The largest section on the pyramid is devoted to foods that are plant-based. Spices, herbs, nuts, olive oil, whole grains, beans, vegetables, and fruits are the most important, and you need to eat these daily. Try to eat seasonal produce and stay away from processed foods if at all possible.

The next section includes seafood and fish. The people of the Mediterranean region normally have fish at least twice each week. Poultry, yogurt, cheese, and eggs are also part of their eating plan, but these are eaten in moderation. Sweets and red meat aren't eaten all that often and are always in very small portions.

You can have a glass of red wine but again in moderation. This is normally only drunk with meals and never more than two glasses per day. Wine can reduce the risk of dementia, boosts the immune system, and improved heart health. Another helpful component of this diet is water. Water is needed for proper digestion and is great for your body.

These components work together to have a great impact on your physical and mental health. They promote the appreciation for delightfully eating tasty and healthy meals. You can also lose some weight with the Mediterranean diet. New research has found that this lifestyle can prevent many diseases. People who followed a Mediterranean diet lost more weight than ones who followed a low-fat diet. These same people had lower waist circumferences, too. The Mediterranean diet can help children either get to a healthy weight or maintain their healthy weight. It can also be beneficial for pregnant women, too.

This is by no means anything new. When most people think Mediterranean they think olive oil and pasta. This is actually a misconception; a normal Mediterranean diet is a prototype of the Cretan diet and contains olive oil, plants, and some carbs here and there. It is a moderately high-fat diet dispersed with some carbs.

If you are looking to lose some weight while following the Mediterranean diet, here are some tips to help you along:

1. Eat your largest meal early

People who live in the Mediterranean region usually eat more at lunchtime. This is normally between one and three in the afternoon. When you move your largest meal to the middle of the day, you are less likely to overeat later in the day. People who eat their largest meal before three will lose more weight.

2. Use vegetables as the main course

Cooking vegetables in olive oil is the magic component of this diet. When you eat vegetables that have been cooked in olive oil, you won't just be satisfied, but you are eating between three to four servings of vegetables at one time. These dishes are low in carbohydrates and have a moderate number of calories. Accompany it with some tomatoes and feta cheese, and you are completely set. Other benefits of eating veggies as your main course are since it isn't a meal rich in carbs, you will avoid being sleepy after you eat.

3. Drink a lot of water

In some countries like the United States, it is normal to drink milk with meals. Is this necessary? No, it isn't. When following the Mediterranean diet, you will get the dairy from yogurt and cheese. Save your calories for solid food instead of liquid calories. This same holds true for juice, too. No one needs juice. You need to eat your fruit. They fill you up, and you also get all the nutrients and fiber. What about wine and coffee? They each have their own place within the diet, but they will not replace water. Greek coffee and red wine give you many health benefits.

4. Eat olive oil in the right amount

Research is continuously confirming what the people from the Mediterranean have known for centuries. Good fats won't make you fat. Yes, calories do count, but in order to stay on a vegetable-based diet, you have to give yourself a variety of flavors but make sure they keep you full. This is what olive oil can do. Olive oil doesn't just make vegetables taste good; it makes them filling. This isn't saying that you need to pour olive oil on everything. A decent amount that will give you the health benefits is around three tablespoons a day.

5. Move

The Mediterranean diet isn't a normal diet; it is a lifestyle, and moving is necessary. Walking is great but moving throughout the day is the main key. It isn't enough to just go to a gym for an hour or two and then go to your place of business and sit for the rest of the day. When you get a break, walk, stand and stretch every hour, clean the house, and if it is feasible, don't drive, walk.

A Mediterranean Kitchen

There isn't one single Mediterranean diet, and there isn't a right or wrong way to follow this diet. The concept brings together all the habits, and common foods from all the traditions in the Mediterranean region and this includes Italy, Portugal, France, Spain, Greece, and Crete. Research is still being done to find the exact benefits of this lifestyle, but it is low in trans fats and free from processed foods, meats, and refined oils. All these items are known to cause cardiovascular disease, cancer, diabetes, and obesity.

Diet Facts

- You need to pair this diet with a lifestyle that is active.

- This diet is high in fats so eating smaller portions and in moderation is recommended.

- This diet can prevent diabetes, protects against stroke, can promote heart health.

- There is a big emphasis on natural sources, lean meats, vegetables, and fruits.

- There isn't just one Mediterranean lifestyle. It contains foods from various countries along the Mediterranean Sea.

Consider this just as a guideline and nothing that is written in stone. This plan is easily adjusted to your preferences and needs.

Basic Foods

Here is a look at the basic foods that are eaten on this diet:

Eat daily: Extra virgin olive oil, seafood, fish, spices, herbs, bread, whole grains, potatoes, legumes, seeds, nuts, fruits, and vegetables.

Moderately: Yogurt, cheese, eggs, and poultry.

Rarely: Red meat.

Never: Very processed foods, refined oils, refined grains, processed meats, added sugars, beverages that have been sweetened with sugar.

Foods to Avoid

Here are some ingredients and foods that you need to avoid:

Highly processed foods: Any foods that are labeled as diet or low fat and that looks like they came from a factory.

Processed meats: hot dogs, sausages, etc.

Refined oil: Cottonseed oil, canola oil, soybean oil.

Trans fats: These are found in processed foods and margarine.

Refined grains: Pasta made from refined wheat, white bread, etc.

Added sugar: Table sugar, ice cream, candy, soda, and many other products.

You have to read labels of foods carefully if you would like to stay away from these ingredients.

What to Eat

The exact foods that belong to the Mediterranean diet are still controversial because there is such a large variation between countries. The diet is known to be high in healthy foods from plants and very low in animal products. It is recommended to eat seafood and fish twice a week. This lifestyle involves regular activity, enjoying life, and sharing meals with loved ones.

You need to base your diet on these healthy foods:

Healthy Fats: avocado oil, avocados, olives, extra virgin olive oil

Spices and Herbs: pepper, cinnamon, nutmeg, sage, rosemary, mint, basil, garlic

Dairy: Greek yogurt, yogurt, cheese

Eggs: Duck, quail, and chicken

Poultry: Turkey, duck, chicken

Seafood and Fish: mussels, crab, clams, oysters, shrimp, mackerel, tuna, trout, sardines, salmon

Whole Grains: whole grain pasta, whole grain bread, whole wheat, buckwheat, corn, barley, rye, brown rice, whole oats

Tubers: yams, turnips, sweet potatoes, potatoes

Legumes: chickpeas, peanuts, pulses, lentils, peas, beans

Seeds and Nuts: pumpkin seeds, sunflower seeds, cashews, hazelnuts, macadamia nuts, walnuts, almonds

Fruits: peaches, melons, figs, dates, grapes, strawberries, pears, oranges, bananas, apples

Vegetables: cucumbers, Brussels sprouts, carrots, cauliflower, onions, spinach, kale, broccoli, tomatoes

Single ingredient, whole foods are the keys to this diet. Since the focus of this diet is on natural sources and plant foods this meant this diet offers nutrients like:

Low sugar: This diet offers natural sugars instead of refined sugar. You get sugar from fresh fruits. Adding in refined sugars will increase calories without giving you any nutritional benefits. This is linked to high blood pressure and diabetes and happens in most of the processed foods that are absent from the Mediterranean lifestyle.

High mineral and vitamin content: Vegetables and fruits give the vital minerals and vitamin that help to regulate our body's processes. Consuming lean meats gives us vitamins like B12 that can't be found in plant foods.

Fiber: A diet that is high in fiber promotes healthy digestion and is thought to reduce the risk of cardiovascular disease and bowel cancer.

Healthful fats: This diet is high in monounsaturated fats and low in saturated fats. Dietary guidelines state that saturated fats shouldn't make up any more than about ten percent of your total calorie intake.

It is hard to give exact nutritional information since there isn't one single diet plan.

What Should You Drink

Water is the main beverage to drink while following the Mediterranean diet. This diet allows you to drink a glass of red wine daily.

This is totally optional, and wine needs to be avoided by anybody who suffers from alcoholism or can't control how much they drink.

Tea and coffee are fine but don't add sugar. If you need cream, use low-fat milk. Stay away from fruit juices and beverages that have been sweetened with sugar. These are super high in sugar.

Here is a normal grocery list to help you get started on your new lifestyle:

Vegetables

- Tomatoes (sauce, canned, fresh)

- Peas

- Kale

- Spinach

- Cabbage

- Artichokes

- Onions

- Broccoli

- Potatoes

- Carrots

- Squash

- Beets

- Sweet potatoes

- Eggplant

- Bell peppers

- Olives

- Garlic

- Mushrooms

- Turnips

- Green beans

- Leeks

- Yams

- Leafy greens (romaine, arugula, swiss chard, collards, mustard greens, etc.)

Fruits
- Pomegranates

- Apples

- Plums

- Apricots

- Peaches

- Avocados

- Oranges

- Bananas

- Melons

- Blueberries

- Lemons

- Cranberries

- Grapes

- Strawberries

- Figs

- Dates

- Cherries

Beans

- Cannellini

- Black beans

- Pinto beans

- Garbanzo

- Lentils

- Pulses

Grains

- Rice

- Barley

- Corn

- Quinoa

- Bulgur

- Polenta

- Buckwheat

- Couscous

- Pasta

- Oatmeal

Spices and Herbs

- Zatar

- Anise

- Thyme

- Basil

- Tarragon

- Bay leaves

- Sumac

- Cilantro

- Savory

- Cumin

- Sage

- Fennel

- Rosemary

- Lavender

- Pul Biber

- Marjoram

- Pepper

- Mint

- Parsley

- Oregano

Seeds and Nuts

- Walnuts

- Almonds

- Sunflower seeds

- Cashews

- Sesame seeds

- Flax

- Pumpkin seeds

- Peanuts

- Pine nuts

Seafood

- Tuna

- Clams

- Tilapia

- Sardines

- Cod

- Shrimp

- Crab

- Scallops

- Oysters

- Salmon

Healthy Fats and Oils

- Grape seed oil

- Avocado oil

- Extra virgin olive oil

- Canola oil

Dairy

- Eggs

- Cheese

- Greek yogurt

- Low-fat milk

- Plain yogurt

Let's take a closer look at some of the main ingredients and how they can help your health:

- Chickpeas

These lovely beans give our body lots of fiber. Fiber protects the body from heart problems, fights diabetes, and reduces the risk of colon cancer. Chickpeas are rich in vitamin K, calcium, zinc, iron, and magnesium. They support strength and bone structure. Vitamin B6 and C can reduce the risk of heart disease.

- Eggplant

Eggplants help protect the body from getting osteoporosis and maintain bone structure. This vegetable doesn't contain any cholesterol or fat. It contains fiber that helps us feel fuller for a longer period. Eggplants can boost brain activity and helps with overall mental health. This is because phytonutrients that increase the blood flow to the brain. This helps improve analytic thoughts and memory.

- Olive oil

This is the main ingredient in the Mediterranean diet, and it brings many health benefits. Oleic acid is the main monounsaturated fatty acid that is found in olive oil. It can suppress the genes that are related to breast cancer. It can also lower inflammation. Olive oil is famous for having strong anti-inflammatory properties. As stated earlier, it can decrease the risk of obesity, Alzheimer's, diabetes, and heart disease. Olive oil can also decrease or destroy harmful bacteria. One of these harmful bacteria is called Helicobacter pylori. This is bacteria located in the stomach that can cause cancer or ulcers.

- Garlic

Garlic is known for being able to boost our immune systems since it contains vitamin C. It also helps reduce the risk of cardiovascular disease by lowering blood pressure.

- Almonds

Eating almonds can boost vitamin E in the red blood cells and plasma. They can also lower cholesterol levels and helps improve heart health. Almonds have a good effect on blood lipids. Eating nuts can reduce breast cancer risk by two to three times.

Recipes

Breakfast

Breakfast Bruschetta

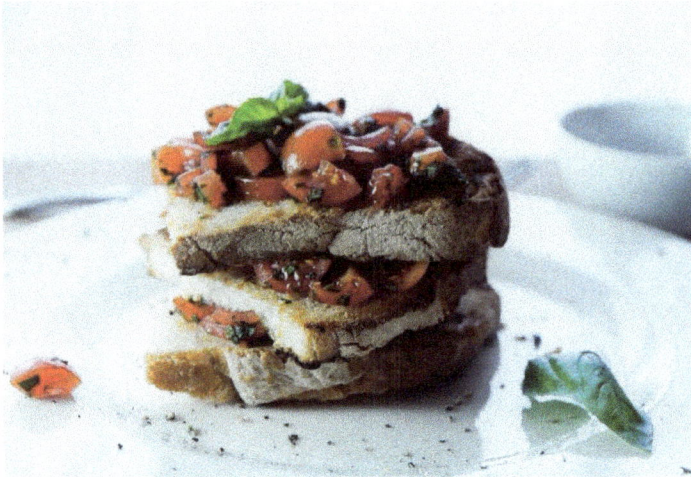

Serves: 4

Sea salt, .25 tsp

¾-inch thick Italian-style whole-grain bread, 4 slices

Halved garlic clove

Grated parmesan, 4 tsp

Pepper, .25 tsp

Milk, 1 tbsp

Eggs, 3

Cooking spray

Crushed red pepper, .25 tsp

½-inch pieces of prosciutto, 1 oz

EVOO, 1 tbsp

Chopped broccoli rabe, 6 c

1. Boil a large pot of water. Add in the broccoli rabe and salt and let the broccoli boil for two minutes. Drain.

2. Add the oil to a large pan and add in the crushed red pepper, prosciutto, and garlic. Cook this for two minutes, stirring frequently. Mix in the broccoli rabe. Cook everything for another three minutes. Pour into a bowl and place to the side.

3. Spritz the pan with the cooking spray and place back over low heat.

4. Beat the pepper, milk, and eggs together. Pour into the pan. Scramble the eggs until they are soft set. This will take about three to five minutes. Add in the broccoli

mixture and the cheese. Cook everything for another minute. Set off the heat.

5. Toast the bread slices and rub them with the garlic halves. You can save the rest of this garlic for later use. Divide the egg mixture between the toast slices and enjoy.

Parsley and Marinara Eggs

Serves: 6

Grated parmesan and crusty Italian bread, for serving – optional

Chopped fresh flat-leaf parsley, .5 c

Eggs, 6

Undrained Italian diced tomatoes, 2 15.4-oz cans

Minced garlic, 2 cloves

Chopped onion, 1 c

EVOO, 1 tbsp

1. Heat the oil up in a large pan. Add in the onion and cook them for about five minutes, stirring often. Mix in the garlic and cook for another minute.

2. Add the tomatoes and their juices into the onion, and cook everything until it starts to bubble. This will take about two to three minutes. While you are waiting on the tomato juices to bubble, break an egg into a custard cup.

3. When the tomato begins bubbling, turn the heat down. With a large spoon, form six indentations in the tomatoes. Carefully pour an egg into an indentation. Crack another egg into the custard cup, and pour it into another indentation. Repeat this process until you have added all of the eggs to your indentations.

4. Place a lid on the pan and cook everything for six to seven minutes or until the eggs are cooked through enough for you.

5. Top the eggs with some parsley and serve with some cheese and bread if you would like.

Goat Cheese and Pepper Eggs

Serves: 4

Loosely packed chopped mint, 2 tbsp

Crumbled goat cheese, .5 c

Water, 2 tbsp

Sea salt, .25 tsp

Eggs, 6

Minced garlic, 2 cloves

Chopped bell peppers, 1 c

EVOO, 1.5 tsp

1. Add the oil to a large pan. Add in the peppers and cook them for five minutes, stirring often. Mix in the garlic and cook everything for a minute.

2. As the peppers cook, beat the water, salt, and eggs together.

3. Lower the heat and add the eggs to the peppers. Allow the eggs to cook, without being touched, for a couple of minutes. Let them set up on the bottom. Top with the goat cheese.

4. Cook for a couple of minutes, stirring slowly until the eggs become soft-set and custard type consistency. They are going to still cook once you take them off the heat.

5. Divide into plates and top with the mint.

Breakfast Bulgur Bowl

Serves: 6

Warm milk, for serving – optional

Chopped loosely packed mint, .25 c

Chopped almonds, .5 c

Chopped figs, 8

Dark sweet cherries, 2 c

Cinnamon, .5 tsp

Water, 1 c

Milk, 2 c

Uncooked bulgur, 1.5 c

1. Add in the cinnamon, water, milk, and bulgur in a pot and mix together. Bring this up to a boil, stirring only once. Place a lid on the pot and let it simmer for ten minutes, or until all of the liquid has been absorbed.

2. Switch off the heat, but keep the pot where it is. Mix in the cherries, almonds, and figs. Place the lid back on and let it sit for a minute. This will partially hydrate dried figs, if you used dried, and thaw the frozen cherries if you used frozen. Mix in the mint.

3. Divide into the bowls and then serve with some warm milk if you want. This can also be served chilled.

Pears and Ricotta

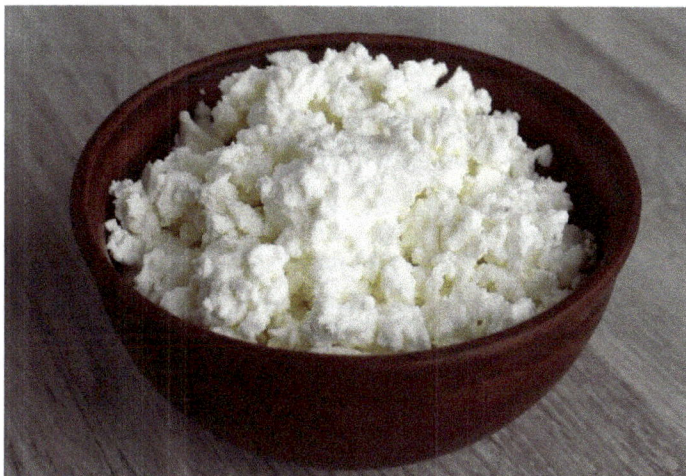

Serves: 4

Honey, 1 tbsp

Water, 2 tbsp

Diced and cored pear

Nutmeg, .25 tsp

Sugar, 1 tbsp

Whole-wheat flour, .25 c

Eggs, 2

Whole-milk ricotta, 16 oz

Cooking spray

1. Start by placing your oven to 400. Grease four 6-ounce ramekins with cooking spray.

2. Beat the nutmeg, vanilla, sugar, flour, eggs, and ricotta together and divide this between the four ramekins. Bake the cheesecakes in your oven for 22-25 minutes, or until it is almost set. Take them out of the oven and set them on cooling racks to cool slightly.

3. As the cheesecakes are baking, add the water and pear to a pot and simmer for ten minutes, or until they are soft. Take them off the heat and mix in the honey.

4. Divide the pear mixture between the tops of the four cheesecakes.

Breakfast Polenta

Serves: 6

Honey, 8 tsp

Greek yogurt, .25 c

Chopped pecans, .5 c

Chopped and peeled oranges, 2

Milk, 2.25 to 2.5 cups – divided

Plain polenta, 2 18-oz tubes

1. Slice the polenta up into rounds and lay them in a microwaveable bowl. Place in the microwave for 45 seconds.

2. Place the polenta in a pot and mash everything up with a fork or potato masher until coarse. Heat this over medium.

3. In another microwavable bowl, heat up the milk for a minute. Go ahead and heat up 2 ½ cups just encase you need the extra ¼ cup. Add two cups of the warmed milk into the polenta and whisk everything together. Continue to mix everything together and mash it up with the whisk. Using the remaining half cup, add in a tablespoon of milk at a time until the polenta becomes fairly smooth and heated. This will take about five minutes. Set this off of the heat.

4. Place the polenta into four bowls and top each with a quarter of an orange, tablespoon of yogurt, two teaspoons of honey, and two tablespoons of pecans. Serve.

Quickie Granola

Serves: 6

Vanilla, 2 tsp

EVOO, .25 c

Honey, .25 c

Ground flaxseed, 2 tbsp

Chopped dried apricots, .5 c

Cinnamon, .5 tsp

Sea salt, pinch

Chopped almonds, .33 c

Rolled oats, 2.5 c

1. Start by placing your oven to 325. Place some parchment on a cooking sheet.

2. Mix in the cinnamon, salt, almonds, and oats together in a large pan. Flip the up to medium-high and cook everything, stirring frequently, for about six minutes. This will toast everything.

3. As the oats are toasting, add the oil, honey, flaxseed, and apricots to a microwavable bowl and cook for a minute, or until it becomes extremely hot and starts to bubble. If you want, you can also heat this in a pot for about three minutes.

4. Mix in the vanilla and then pour the mixture over the oats in the pan. Mix everything together.

5. Spread the oat mixture out on the cooking sheet. Bake the granola for about 15 minutes, or until it becomes browned. Take this out of the oven and let it cool completely.

6. Break it up into smaller pieces and keep in an airtight container. It should stay refrigerated and will last for about two weeks. This can be served on top of some Greek yogurt or eaten on its own.

Mediterranean Avocado Toast

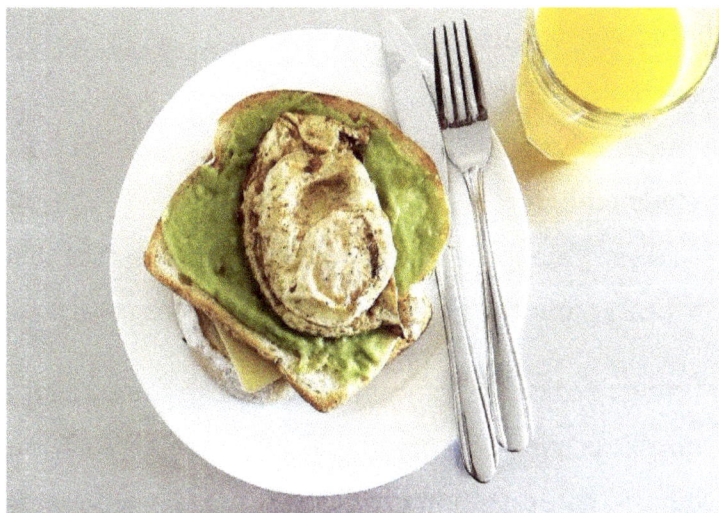

Serves: 4

Avocado

Rinsed and drained chickpeas, 15 oz can

Honey, 2 tsp

Multigrain toast, 4 slices

Pepper, .5 tsp

Lemon juice, 2 tsp

Diced feta cheese, .5 c

1. Add the chickpeas to a bowl. Scoop the flesh of the avocado into the bowl with the chickpeas.

2. Using a fork or a potato masher, mash them together until it becomes a spreadable consistency. You don't have to get it completely smooth.

3. Mix in the pepper, lemon juice, and feta.

4. Divide the mixture between four toast slices. Drizzle with some honey and enjoy.

Green Pasta

Serves: 4

Honey, 4 tsp

Chopped walnuts, .5 c

Greek yogurt, 2 c

EVOO, 1 tbsp

Seedless grapes, 1.5 lb

1. Start by placing your oven to 450. Slide a large cooking sheet in the oven to preheat.

2. Wash off the grapes and get rid of their stem. Lay them on a kitchen towel to dry them off. Add them to a bowl and toss with the oil.

3. Carefully take the cooking sheet out of the oven and lay the grapes on the sheet. Bake them for 20-23 minutes, or until they have shriveled up a bit. Stir them halfway through the cooking process. Take this out of the oven and place them on the wire rack to cool for five minutes.

4. As the grapes cool, place the yogurt in the bottom of four tall glasses or bowls. Tops each of these with a teaspoon of honey and two tablespoons of walnuts.

5. Once the grapes have cooled off slightly, top each one of the parfaits with a quarter of the grapes. Make sure you

divide any of the accumulated juices between the parfaits. Enjoy.

Smoothie Bowl

Serves: 4

Pomegranate juice, .75 c

Greek yogurt, 1.5 c – more if you need it

Frozen dark sweet cherries, 16 oz bag

Pomegranate seeds, .5 c

Chopped pistachios, .5 c

Ice cubes, 6

Cinnamon, .75 tsp

Vanilla, 1 tsp

Milk, .33 c – more if you need it

1. Place the ice cubes, cinnamon, vanilla, milk, pomegranate juice, yogurt, and cherries in a blender. Mix everything together until smooth. The mixture needs to be thicker than your average smoothie. Thicker than would be able to be sucked up through a straw but not so thick that you can't pour it. If you find that it is too thick, add in some more milk. Add in some more yogurt if it is too thin.

2. Divide the smoothie between four bowls and top each with two tablespoons of pomegranate seeds and two tablespoons of pistachios and enjoy.

Egg and Yogurt Oatmeal

Servings 1

Sugar to taste

Salt to taste

Diced apple, .25 c

Yogurt, .25 c

Cinnamon, .25 tsp

Egg, 1

Low-fat milk, .33 c

Oats, .33 c

1. Crack the egg into a microwave safe bowl and add milk. Whisk until blended.

2. Add remaining ingredients except for the apple and yogurt and stir to combine.

3. Place in microwave and cook two minutes or until liquid is absorbed.

4. Add the apples and yogurt to the top and enjoy.

Spinach and Egg Bake

Servings 4

Chunky salsa, .25 c

Shredded cheddar, 25 c

Chopped, thawed, frozen spinach, 1 pkg

Eggs, 4

1. You need to warm your oven to 325.

2. Divide the spinach equally into four ramekins. Press your fingers into the spinach to make a well.

3. Crack an egg in each ramekin. Add cheese and salsa to the top.

4. Place all ramekins on a baking sheet. Put into oven for 20 minutes.

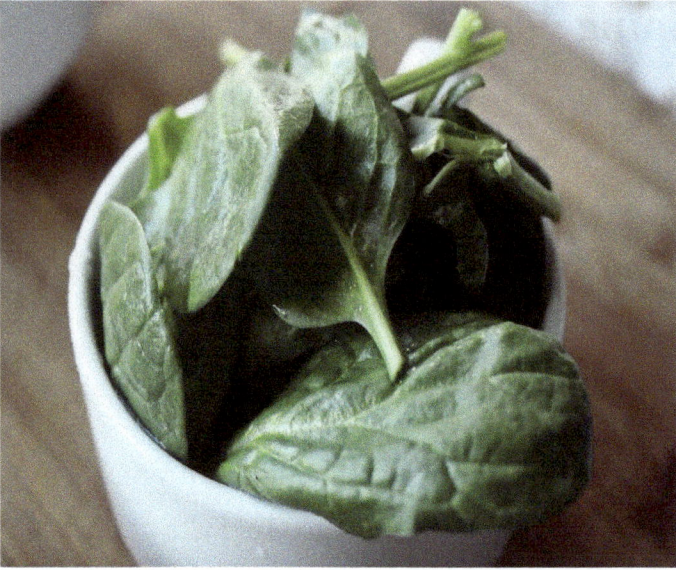

Fruity Quinoa

Servings 4

Cinnamon, 1 tsp

Large dried figs, 4

Halved dried apricots, 8

Walnuts, .25 c

Rinsed quinoa, 1 c

Water, 3 c

1. Add water and quinoa to a pot and bring to a simmer.

2. Let simmer 15 minutes or until all water has been absorbed.

3. Chop the dried fruit.

4. Once the quinoa has cooked, add in fruit and stir well.

5. Add milk, if desired.

6. Can be eaten warm or cold.

Cheese and Eggs Hash

Servings 1

Pepper, to taste

Salt, to taste

Feta cheese, 2 tbsp

Frozen shredded hash browns, .5 c

Egg, 1

1. Spray a microwave-safe bowl with olive oil cooking spray. Add in hash browns.

2. Place in microwave for one minute. Carefully remove from microwave.

3. Add pepper and salt to taste. Crack in an egg and mix well.

4. Place into the microwave for another 45 seconds.

5. Carefully remove from microwave and sprinkle on cheese.

Veggie Bowl

Servings 1

Sliced cherry tomatoes, 2

Chopped baby spinach, 25 c

Diced mushrooms, 2

Shredded mozzarella, .25 c

Water, 1 tbsp

Egg, 1

1. Crack the egg into a microwave safe bowl add in remaining ingredients except for the cheese. Whisk until blended.

2. Place in microwave and cook one minute or until egg is cooked to your liking.

3. Sprinkle on cheese and enjoy.

Lunch

Fagioli Soup

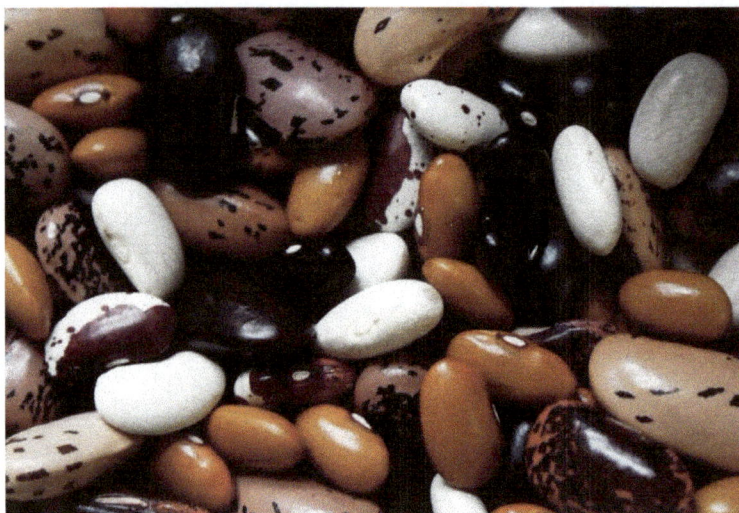

Serves: 6

Grated parmesan, 6 tbsp

Uncooked short pasta, 8 oz

Tomato paste, 2 tbsp

Low-sodium crush tomatoes, 28 oz can

Undrained cannellini, light kidney, or great northern beans, 2 15.5-oz cans

Low-sodium vegetable broth, 4 c

Crushed red pepper, .25 tsp

Dried rosemary, 1 tsp

Minced garlic, 3 cloves

Chopped onion, .5 c

EVOO, 2 tbsp

1. Add the oil to a large pot. Add in the onion and cook them for around four minutes, stirring often. Mix in the crushed red pepper, rosemary, and garlic. Cook for another minute, stirring often. Pour in the broth, along with the tomato paste, tomatoes, and the beans with their liquid. Simmer all of this for five minutes.

2. To make the soup thicker, pour two cups of the soup to a blender and puree. Pour this back into the pot of soup.

3. Allow all of this to come up to a boil. Stir in the pasta and then lower the heat back down. Cook the soup until the pasta is cooked through. Stir every few minutes to make sure that the pasta doesn't stick. Bite into a piece of pasta to make sure that it is cooked. It may need to take a few minutes longer than what is recommended on the box.

4. Ladle into bowls and top with a tablespoon of cheese.

Greek Salad Wraps

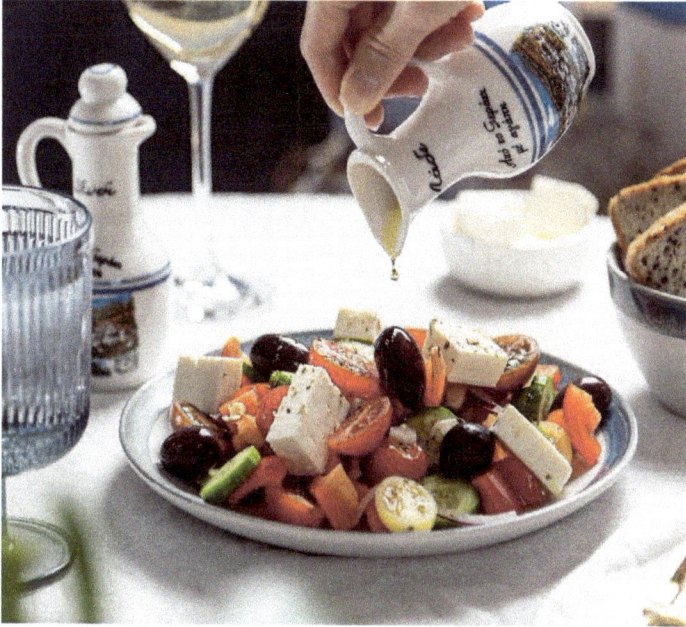

Serves: 4

Drained sliced black olives, .5 c

Chopped fresh mint, .5 c

Chopped tomato, 1 c

Chopped and peeled seedless cucumber, 1.5 c

Whole-wheat flatbread wraps, 4

Crumbled goat cheese, .5 c

Sea salt, .25 tsp

Pepper, .25 tsp

Red wine vinegar, 1 tbsp

EVOO, 2 tbsp

Diced red onion, .25 c

1. Stir together the onion, olives, mint, tomato, and cucumber until well mixed.

2. Beat the salt, pepper, vinegar, and oil together. Drizzle this over the cucumber mixture and toss everything together.

3. Spread the goat cheese across the wraps and spoon in a quarter of the salad across the center of the wraps.

4. To fold up the wraps, fold the bottom edge up and then fold one side over, followed by the other side. Repeat with the other wraps.

Green Pasta

Serves: 4

Grated Pecorino Romano, .33 c

Sliced green olives, .33 c

Sea salt, .25 tsp

Pepper, .25 tsp

Nutmeg, .25 tsp

Loosely packed baby spinach, 5 c

Chopped flat-leaf parsley, 2 c

Crushed red pepper, .25 tsp

Minced garlic, 2 cloves

EVOO, 1 tbsp

Uncooked penne, 8 oz

6. Cook the penne according to the directions on the package, but cook it for a minute less than the instructions say to. Drain off the paste and reserve a quarter cup of the water.

7. As the pasta is cooking, heat the oil in a large pan. Add in the crushed red pepper and garlic and let this cook for 30 seconds, constantly stirring. Mix in the parsley and cook for another minute, still constantly stirring. Stir in the salt, pepper, nutmeg, and spinach. Cook this for three minutes, stirring often, until the spinach has wilted.

8. Mix the pasta and the reserved water into the pan. Mix in the olives and cook for two minutes, or until the majority of the water has been absorbed by the pasta. Take this off the heat and mix in the cheese. Serve.

Paella Soup

Serves: 6

Cleaned medium shrimp, 1 lb

Low-sodium crushed tomatoes, 28 oz

Water, 2.5 c

Low-sodium chicken broth, 2 c

Uncooked instant brown rice, 2.5 c

Smoked paprika, 2 tsp

Dried thyme, 1 tsp

Turmeric, 1 tsp

Chopped garlic, 2 cloves

Chopped green bell pepper, 1.5 c

Chopped red bell pepper, 1.5 c

Chopped onion, 1 c

EVOO, 2 tbsp

Frozen green peas, 1 c

1. Place the peas on a counter so that they will thaw as you prepare the soup.

2. Heat the oil in a large pot. Cook the garlic, bell peppers, and onion together. Cook all of the veggies for eight minutes, stirring often. Mix in the smoked paprika, thyme, and turmeric. Cook everything for two more minutes, stirring often. Mix in the water, broth, and

rice. Let this come up to a boil. Place on the lid and then lower the heat down to a simmer. Let this cook for ten minutes.

3. Mix in the shrimp, tomatoes, and peas. Cook for four to six minutes more, or until the shrimp is cooked. The shrimp should be pink when done. The soup should be almost a stew-like consistency. Enjoy.

Carrot Soup with Croutons

Serves: 4

Grated parmesan, .33 c

Whole-grain bread, 4 slices

Sea salt, .25 tsp

Crushed red pepper, .25 tsp

Dried thyme, 1 tsp

Water, 2.5 c

Low-sodium vegetable broth, 2 c

Chopped onion, 1 c

EVOO, 2 tbsp – divided

½-inch thick sliced carrots, 2 lb

1. Place the rack in your oven about four inches under the broiler. Set your oven to 450. Place two large cooking sheets in your oven.

2. Toss the carrots in a tablespoon of oil. Using oven mitts, take out the cooking sheets and evenly place the carrots on the two cooking sheets. Place them back in the oven and cook for 20 minutes, or until the carrots have become fork tender. Make sure you stir them about halfway through. They will still be a little bit firm. Take the carrots out of the oven and then switch the oven to broil.

3. As the carrots are roasting, add a tablespoon of oil to a large pot and cook the onions. Cook them for five minutes, occasionally stirring. Mix in the salt, crushed red pepper, thyme, water, and broth. Allow this all to come up to a boil and place on the lid. Take the pan off of the heat until the carrots of roasted.

4. Mix the carrots into the pot and then use an immersion blender to mix the soup until smooth. If an immersion blender isn't available, you can carefully blend the soup up in a blender until smooth. Make sure you are careful when you do this. Add everything back in the pot and heat everything through again.

5. Lay the bread on a cooking sheet and top the bread with the cheese. Broil the toast for a couple of minutes, or until the cheese has completely melted. Make sure you watch it so that it doesn't end up burning.

6. Slice the bread into croutons. Pour the soup into separate bowls and top them with the croutons. Enjoy.

Barley Mushroom Soup

Serves: 6

Grated parmesan, 6 tbsp

Bay leaf

Dried thyme, .5 tsp

Tomato paste, 2 tbsp

Red wine, .25 c

Uncooked pearled barley, 1 c

Low-sodium vegetable broth, 6 c

Chopped mushrooms, 5.5 c

Chopped carrots, 1 c

Chopped onion, 1 c

EVOO, 2 tbsp

1. Heat the oil in a large pot. Cook the carrots and the onion for about five minutes, stirring often. Up the heat and mix in the mushrooms. Cook everything for three minutes more, stirring often.

2. Mix in the bay leaf, thyme, tomato paste, wine, barley, and broth. Stir everything together and place the lid on the pot. Let everything come to a boil. Once it starts to boil, stir it a few times, and then turn the heat down. Keeping it covered, cook for 12-15 minutes more, or until the barley is cooked.

3. Take the bay leaf out of the soup and divide between bowls. Top each with a tablespoon of cheese.

Chicken Soup

Serves: 6

Grated parmesan, 3 tbsp

Shredded cooked chicken, 2 c

Uncooked acini de pepe, .75 c

Pepper, .25 tsp

Sea salt, .25 tsp

Low-sodium chicken broth, 8 c

Minced carrots, 1 c

Packed chopped kale, 3 c

Minced garlic, 2 cloves

EVOO, 1 tbsp

1. Heat the oil in a large pot. Add in the garlic, cooking for 30 seconds. Mix in the carrots and kale, and cook for another five minutes, stirring often.

2. Stir in the pepper, salt, and broth. Switch the heat to high and let everything start to boil. Mix in the pasta. Turn the heat down and cook everything for ten minutes or until the pasta has cooked. Stir every so often so that the pasta doesn't stick to the bottom of the pot. Mix in the chicken and cook for two more minutes.

3. Divide the soup into bowls and top each one of them with ½ tablespoon of cheese.

Panzanella Salad

Serves: 4

Fresh chopped oregano and grated parmesan, for serving – option

Sea salt, .25 tsp

Pepper, .5 tsp

Balsamic vinegar, 1 tbsp

Cubed whole-grain crusty bread, 3 c

Honey, 1.5 tsp – divided

Cherry tomatoes, 1 pint

EVOO, 3 tbsp – divided

Broccoli florets, 1 lb

1. Start by placing your oven to 450. Place a large baking sheet in the oven to heat up.

2. Toss the broccoli florets in a tablespoon of oil. Make sure that it is well coated.

3. Carefully take the baking sheet out of the oven and spread the broccoli out onto the tray. Make sure some of the oil stays in the bottom of the bowl. Place the tomatoes in the bowl and toss them in the leftover oil, don't add in any extra oil. Add in a teaspoon of honey and toss the tomatoes again. Scrap this onto the tray with the broccoli.

4. Place in the oven and cook for 15 minutes, stirring once. Take the tray out of the oven and top with the bread cubes. Rose for another three minutes. Once the broccoli is slightly charred and is fork tender, it is done.

5. Place the veggies onto a serving platter.

6. Beat the remaining oil with the vinegar and remaining honey. Add in some salt and pepper. Pour this over the vegetables and toss everything together. Top with some oregano and cheese if you want and enjoy.

Potato Salad

Serves: 6

Torn mint, 2 tbsp

Chopped oregano, 2 tbsp

Sliced celery, 1 c

Sliced olive, .5 c

Sea salt, .25 tsp

Olive brine, 1 tbsp

EVOO, 3 tbsp

Lemon juice, 3 tbsp

Yukon Gold baby potatoes, 2 lbs – cut into 1-inch cubes

1. Cover the potatoes with water in a pot and bring the water to a boil. Lower the heat and let them simmer for 12-15 minutes. The potatoes should be fork tender.

2. As the potatoes cook, beat together the salt, olive brine, oil, and lemon juice.

3. Drain the water from the potatoes and place them in a serving bowl. Immediately add three tablespoons of the dressing on the potatoes. Carefully mix in the celery and olives.

4. Before you serve, add in the rest of the dressing, mint, and oregano.

Antipasto Salad

Serves: 6

Salad –

Sliced black olives, .5 c

Cubed feta cheese, .5 c

Chopped and peeled cucumber

Halved grape tomatoes, 1 pint

Halved and drained artichoke hearts, 14 oz

Rinsed and drained chickpeas, 15 oz

Loosely packed chopped basil, .25 c

Bibb lettuce, 1 head

Dressing –

Pepper, .25 tsp

Honey, 1 tsp

Chopped fresh oregano, 1 tbsp

Lemon juice, 1 tbsp

Red wine vinegar, 1 tbsp

EVOO, 3 tbsp

1. To make the salad – Chop the lettuce and toss it together with the basil. Spread this across a serving plate or in a bowl. Place the olives, feta, cucumber, tomatoes, artichoke hearts, and chickpeas over the top of the lettuce layer.

2. To make the dressing – Beat together the pepper, honey, oregano, lemon juice, vinegar, and oil. The

dressing can be served on the side, or you can drizzle the dressing over the salad.

Melon Caprese

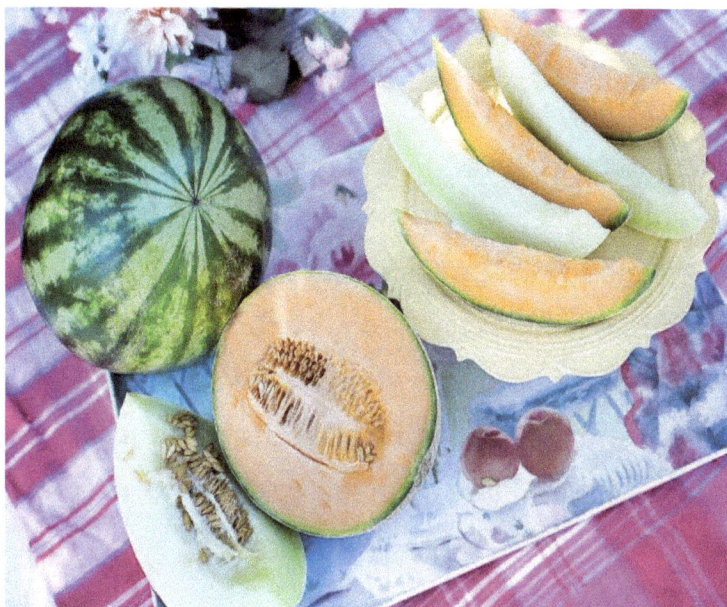

Serves: 6

Sea salt, .25 tsp

Pepper, .25 tsp

Balsamic vinegar, 1 tbsp

EVOO, 2 tbsp

Torn basil, .33 c

Fresh mozzarella balls, 2 c

Grape tomatoes, 1 c

Small seedless watermelon, .5

Quartered and seeded cantaloupe

1. Using a melon baller, scoop out balls of the cantaloupe. You should be able to get about 2 ½ to 3 cups. If you don't want to fool with make balls, you can cut them into squares. Place them in a colander set over top of a serving bowl.

2. Do the same thing with the watermelon. This should give you about two cups. Place the watermelon balls in the colander with the cantaloupe.

3. Allow the fruit to sit like this for ten minutes. The juice that is left in the bowl can be poured into a container and kept in the fridge for smoothies or for drinking. Clean out the bowl and add in the fruit.

4. Add the salt, pepper, vinegar, oil, basil, mozzarella, and tomatoes to the fruit. Carefully toss everything together so that it is well incorporated. Enjoy.

Celery and Orange Salad

Serves: 6

Sliced celery, 3 stalks

Pepper, .25 tsp

Sea salt, .25 tsp

Orange juice, 1 tbsp

Olive brine, 1 tbsp

EVOO, 1 tbsp

Sliced red onion, .25 c

Green olives, .5 c

Peeled and sliced orange, 2

1. Lay the onion, olives, oranges, and celery into a wide bowl.

2. Beat together the orange juice, olive brine, and oil. Pour the dressing over the salad and top with some pepper and salt. Enjoy.

Pistachio and Arugula Salad

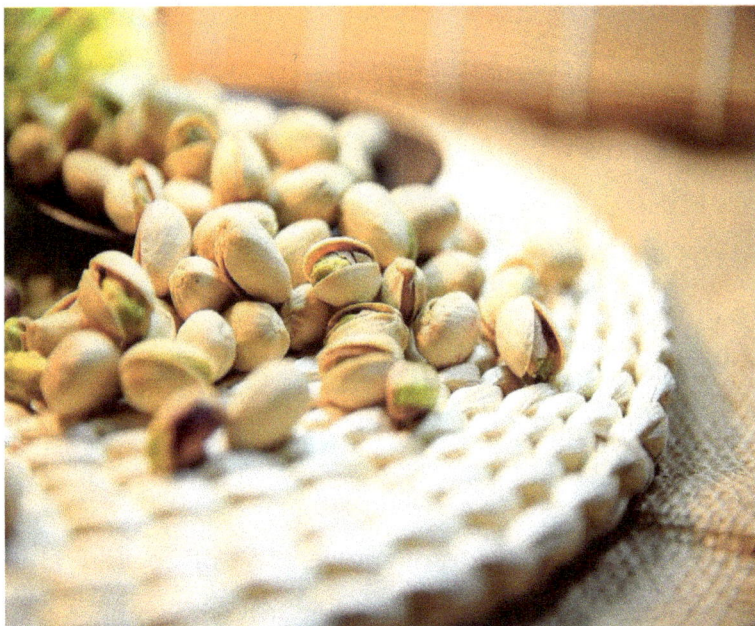

Serves: 6

EVOO, .25 c

Chopped kale, 6 c

Grated parmesan, 6 tbsp

Unsalted shelled pistachios, .33 c

Arugula, 2 c

Smoked paprika, .5 tsp

Lemon juice, 2 tbsp

1. Add the smoked paprika, lemon juice, oil, and kale in a large bowl. Using your hands, massage the kale leaves for around 15 seconds, or until they are all coated. Allow the kale to sit for about ten minutes. This will ensure that the kale is easier to eat.

2. Once you are ready to enjoy the salad, carefully mix in the pistachios and arugula. Place the salad into bowls and top each with a tablespoon of grated cheese. Enjoy.

Chicken Wraps

Serves: 6

Loosely packed chopped flat-leaf parsley, 1.5 c

Sliced mozzarella, 1 c

Whole-wheat spinach wraps, 6 8-in

Dried oregano, 1 tsp

Low-sodium crushed tomatoes, 1 c

Garlic powder, .75 tsp – divided

Grated parmesan, .5 c

Whole-wheat panko, .66 c

Buttermilk, .25 c

Egg

Skinless, boneless chicken breasts, 1 lb

Cooking spray

1. Start by placing your oven to 425. Place some foil on a baking sheet. Lay a rack on the foil-lined baking sheet and spray everything with cooking spray. Set to the side.

2. Place the chicken in a bag and use a rolling pin or mallet to beat the chicken so that it is evenly flat. You want to get to about a quarter inch thick. Slice into six pieces. You may have to put two smaller pieces together to get the sixth piece.

3. Beat the buttermilk and eggs together in a shallow bowl. In a different bowl, place the panko breadcrumbs, half teaspoon of garlic powder, and the parmesan. Dip each portion into the egg wash and then into the panko mixture. Press the crumbs into the chicken to make sure that they stick. Lay the chicken on your wire rack.

4. Bake this for 15-18 minutes, or until it reaches 165. All of the juices should run clear. Place the chicken on a cutting board and slice into ½-inch pieces.

5. Combine the remaining garlic powder, oregano, and tomatoes in a microwavable bowl. Place a paper towel over the bowl and microwave for a minute. Place to the side.

6. Wrap the tortillas with a damp towel and microwave for 30-45 seconds.

7. To make the wraps, place the chicken slices on the six tortillas and top them with the cheese. Add a tablespoon of the tomato sauce over everything and then sprinkle each with ¼ cup of parsley. To wrap up the tortilla, fold the bottom up, and then fold in one side followed by the other. Serve with any of the remaining sauce for dipping.

Salmon Salad Wrap

Serves: 6

Whole-wheat flatbread wraps, 4

Sea salt, .25 tsp

Pepper, .5 tsp

Balsamic vinegar, 1 tbsp

EVOO, 1.5 tbsp

Capers, 2 tbsp

Diced red onion, 3 tbsp

Chopped dill, 3 tbsp

Diced celery, .5 c

Diced carrots, .5 c

Cooked and flaked salmon, 1 lb

1. Mix together the salt, pepper, vinegar, oil, capers, red onion, dill, celery, carrots, and salmon.

2. Split the salmon salad between the flatbread wraps. Fold up the bottom and then roll the wrap-up and enjoy.

Falafels

Serves: 4

Medium tomato cut into four slices

Whole-wheat pitas, 2 – cut in half

Minced garlic clove

Greek yogurt, 6 oz

Cucumber sliced in half lengthwise

EVOO, 1 tbsp

Pepper, .25 tsp

Dried oregano, 2 tsp

Egg

Whole-wheat panko, .5 c

Hummus, .5 c

Rinsed and drained chickpeas, 15 oz can

1. Mash up the chickpeas with a fork or potato masher until it is still somewhat chunky. Add in the hummus, pepper, oregano, egg, and panko. Mix everything together until combined. Using your hands, form the chickpea mixture into four patties. They should be ½ cup size. Press them out to ¾ inch thickness and place on a plate.

2. Add the oil to a large pan and heat until very hot. This will take about three minutes. Place the patties in the pan and cook them for five minutes on both sides.

3. As the patties cook, shred half the cucumber using a box grater. You can also chop it up finely with a knife. Mix together the garlic, yogurt, and shredded cucumber to make your tzatziki sauce. Slice up the other half of the cucumber and place to the side.

4. Toast your pita bread. To make your sandwich, place a pita half on a plate. Inside the pita, add a few cucumber slices, a patty, and a slice of tomato. Add in some tzatziki sauce and enjoy.

Veggie Panini

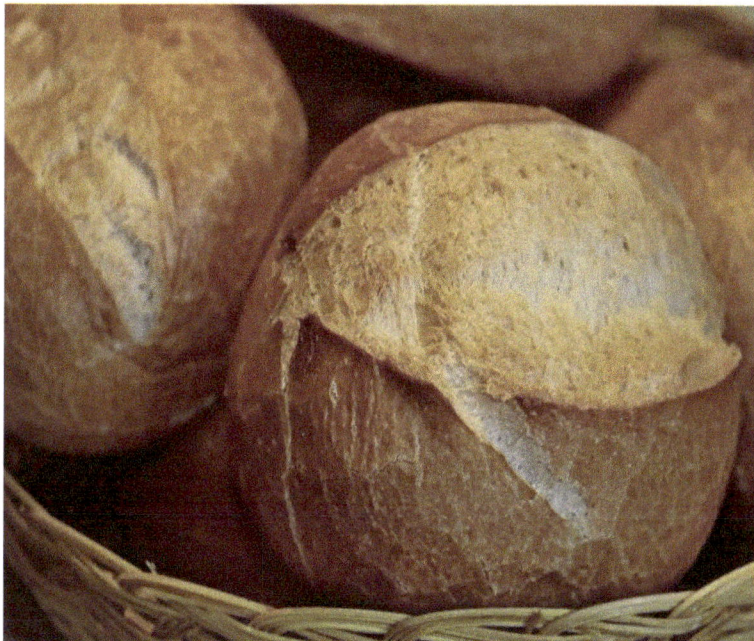

Serves: 4

2-foot-long whole-grain Italian loaf sliced in fourths

Sliced mozzarella, 1 c

Grated parmesan, 2 tbsp

Drained and chopped roasted red peppers, 12 oz jar

Cooking spray

Sea salt, pinch

Pepper, pinch

Dried oregano, .25

Diced onion, .25 c

Diced zucchini, 1 c

Diced broccoli, 1.5 c

EVOO, 2 tbsp - divided

1. Start by placing your oven to 450. Place a large cooking tray in the oven to heat up.

2. Combine the salt, pepper, oregano, onion, zucchini, broccoli, and a tablespoon of oil together.

3. Take the baking tray out of the oven, and carefully spray it with some cooking spray. Spread the veggies across the ban and cook for five minutes. Stir them once during the cooking time.

4. Take the tray out of the oven and add on the parmesan and red peppers and stir everything together.

5. Using either a large pan, grill pan, or Panini maker, heat up the rest of the oil.

6. Slice open a section of the bread but don't slice all the way through. Add a half cup of the veggies onto the bread and top with an ounce of the mozzarella cheese. Close up the sandwich and place two sandwiches on your pan, grill, or Panini press.

7. If using a Panini press, close and grill the sandwich for three to five minutes or until it had a good crust and the cheese melts. With a pan or grill, lay a heavy object on the sandwich and grill for 2 ½ minutes, flip and cook for another 2 ½ minutes.

8. Repeat this process for the rest of the sandwiches.

Margherita Sandwiches

Serves: 4

Pepper, .25 tsp

Lightly packed torn basil, .25 c

Sliced mozzarella, 1 c

Dried oregano, .25 tsp

Large tomato sliced into 8 slices

Halved garlic clove

EVOO, 1 tbsp

Whole-wheat hoagie rolls, 2 – sliced open

1. Heat up your broiler and place the topmost rack to about four inches under the element.

2. Lay the bread out on a baking sheet. Lay the bread under the broil for a minute, or until it has toasted lightly. Be very careful to make sure that it doesn't burn. Take it out of the oven.

3. Brush the bread with some oil and rub with the garlic.

4. While still on the baking sheet, distribute the tomato slices on each piece. Sprinkle them with oregano and top it with the cheese.

5. Place this back under the broiler and let this cook for a minute. Keep an eye on it. Once the cheese has melted

and the edges have started to brown, take them out of the oven.

6. Top with some fresh cracked pepper and basil.

Tuna Sandwich

Serves: 4

EVOO, 2 tbsp

Lemon juice, 3 tbsp

Whole-grain crusty bread, 8 slices

Chopped fennel, .5 c

Slice olives, .5 c

Drained tuna, 2 5-oz cans

Pepper, .5 tsp

Minced garlic clove

1. Mix together the pepper, garlic, oil, and lemon juice. Add the fennel, olives, and tune to the dressing. Using a fork, break apart the tuna and mix everything together.

2. Divide the tuna salad on top of four bread slices. Lay the remaining bread slices on top. Allow the sandwiches to rest for five minutes. This will allow the filling and juices to soak into the bread. Enjoy.

Prosciutto Avocado Sandwich

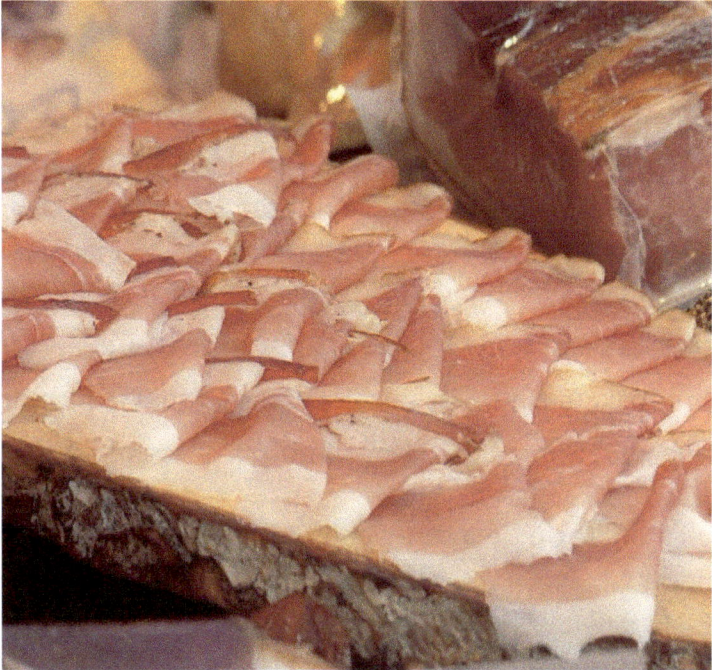

Serves: 4

Prosciutto, 2 oz – sliced into 8 slices

Large tomato sliced into 8 rounds

Romaine leaves, 4 torn into 8 pieces

Sea salt, .25 tsp

Pepper, .25 tsp

Avocado

Whole-grain bread, 8 slices

1. Toast the slices of bread and then lay them on a plate.

2. Scoop the flesh out of the avocado into a small bowl. Sprinkle in some salt and pepper. With either a whisk or fork, mash up the avocado until it makes a creamy spread. Spread this over the slices of bread.

3. To finish up the sandwiches, take a slice of toast and add on a lettuce leaf, prosciutto slice, and a slice of tomato. Then lay on another lettuce leaf, prosciutto slice, and tomato. Top with the second piece of avocado toast. Do to make the three remaining sandwiches. Enjoy.

Pasta Salad with Avocado

Servings 6

Sliced onion, 3

Cooked pasta, 4 c

Chopped red bell pepper, 1

Diced avocado, 1

Dijon mustard, 2 tsp

White wine vinegar, 1 tbsp

Segments from 2 oranges

EVOO, 1.5 tbsp

Orange juice, .33 c

Marmalade, 3 tbsp

1. Place the vinegar, oil, mustard, marmalade, and juice into a bowl and mix well until blended.

2. Add in the pasta and place in the refrigerator for one hour.

3. When ready to serve, mix in remaining ingredients and enjoy.

Cretan Salad

Servings 4

Cubed Feta cheese, 4 oz

Lemon juice, .5 c

Greek olives, .5 c

Sliced onion, 1

Sliced tomatoes, 2

Sliced cucumbers, 2

Sliced zucchinis, 2

Hard boiled eggs, 3

Cubed potatoes, 4

1. Place the zucchini and potatoes into a pot of boiling water and boil until fork tender. Drain and allow to cool completely.

2. Cut the hardboiled eggs into wedges.

3. Add all of the ingredients to a bowl. Stir to mix well. Season with pepper and salt. Enjoy.

Smoked Salmon Sandwiches

Servings 4 to 8

Fresh dill sprigs

Baby spinach leaves

Sliced cucumber, 1

Smoked salmon, 4 oz

Feta cheese, .25 c

Whole grain rolls, 4

1. Slice the rolls in half. Place them side by side on the counter.

2. Evenly distribute the cheese onto one half of each roll.

3. Place some baby spinach leaves, dill, cucumber, and salmon on top of the cheese.

4. You can either eat one whole roll or cut in half and eat a smaller portion.

Lentil Soup

Servings 6

Pepper to taste

Salt to taste

Tomato paste, 2 tbsp

Segments of one orange

Minced garlic, 2 cloves

Grated carrots, 3

Grated onion, 1

EVOO, 1 c

Water, 6 c

Lentils, 1 lb

1. Rinse the lentils under running water and remove any stones or debris.

2. Place into a pot with the water and boil 15 minutes.

3. Add in remaining ingredients and continue to cook for 30 minutes.

4. Taste and adjust seasoning as needed.

5. Ladle into soup bowls and enjoy.

Strawberry Salad

Servings 6

Candied walnuts, .5 c

Crumbled blue cheese, .5 c

Chopped pitted dried dates, .5 c

Quartered strawberries, 1 c

Lettuce, 5 oz

Sliced Kalamata olives, 1 c

1. Divide the lettuce onto six salad plates.

2. Divide the remaining ingredients on top of the lettuce and serve.

Dinner

Shrimp Puttanesca

Serves: 4

Cleaned shrimp, 1 lb

Chopped fresh oregano, 1 tbsp

Capers, 2 tbsp

Drained sliced black olives, .5 c

Low-sodium diced tomatoes, 14.5 oz can – undrained

Crushed red pepper, .5 tsp

Minced garlic, 3 cloves

Anchovy paste, 1.5 tsp

EVOO, 2 tbsp

1. Heat the oil in a large pan. Stir in the crushed red pepper, garlic, and anchovies. Cook everything for about three minutes, stirring often. Mash up the anchovies, until they are melted into the olive oil.

2. Mix in the oregano, capers, olives, and the tomatoes and their juices. Up the heat so that everything starts to simmer.

3. Once the sauce starts to bubble a bit, mix in the shrimp. Lower the heat back down and let the shrimp cook for six to eight minutes, or until the shrimp turn pink and

white. Stir occasionally. Once the shrimp is cooked,
serve.

Cauliflower Steaks

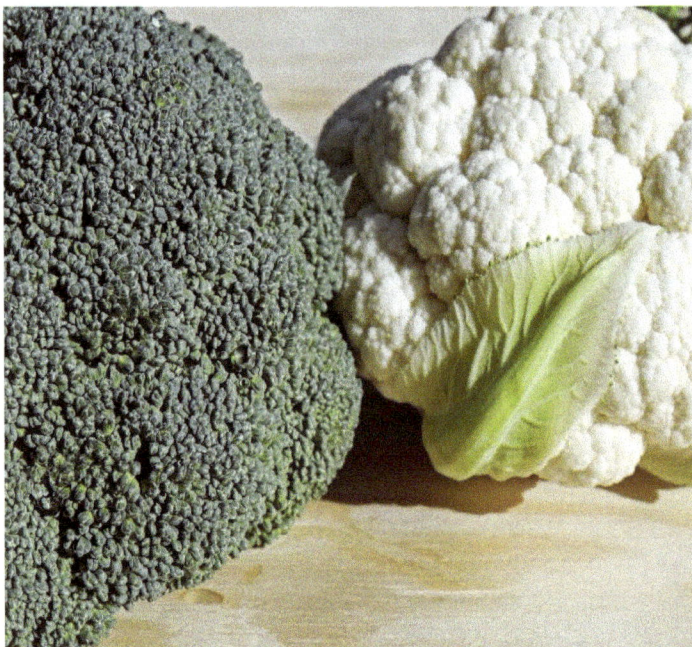

Serves: 4

Baba ghanoush, 1 container

EVOO

Smoked paprika, .25 tsp

Sea salt, .25 tsp

Cauliflower, 2 small heads

1. Start by setting your oven to 400 and place a large baking sheet in the oven to get hot.

2. Place a head of cauliflower with the stem-side down on a cutting board. Using a large knife, slice through the center of the head of cauliflower. On both halves of the cauliflower, slice off a one-inch thick steak. Reserve the rest of the cauliflower for later use. Do the same with the second head of cauliflower.

3. Dry of the steaks and sprinkle them with paprika and salt on both sides.

4. Add two tablespoons of oil to a large pan. Once the oil is smoking hot, place two cauliflowers steaks in and cook them for three minutes, or until crispy. Flip, and cook another two minutes. Place the steaks on a plate. Hold a paper towel with some tongs and wipe out the pan to get rid of the oil. Using the remaining oil, repeat this cooking process with the remaining steaks.

5. Carefully take the baking sheet out of the oven using oven mitts. Place the cauliflower steaks on the hot baking sheet. It will sizzle when you do this. Roast the steaks for 12-15 minutes, or until the steaks become fork tender. You still want them to be a bit firm. You don't want your steak to be mush. Serve your cauliflower steaks with some baba ghanoush.

Shrimp Gnocchi Bake

Serves: 4

Torn fresh basil, .33 c

Cubed feta, .5 c

Frozen gnocchi, 1 lb

Cleaned fresh shrimp, 1 lb

Chopped roasted red peppers, 12 jar

Crushed red pepper, .25 tsp

Pepper, .5 tsp

Minced garlic, 2 cloves

EVOO, 2 tbsp

Chopped tomato, 1 c

1. Start by placing your oven to 425.

2. Using a casserole dish, combine the crushed red pepper, pepper, garlic, oil, and tomatoes. Bake this for ten minutes.

3. Once the roasting time is up, add in the shrimp and roasted peppers. Roast this for another ten minutes or until it turns opaque

4. As the shrimp is baking, cook your gnocchi according to the directions on the package. Drain off the gnocchi and keep warm.

5. Take the casserole from the oven and stir in the basil, feta, and gnocchi. Enjoy.

Garlic Shrimp

Serves: 6

Cleaned fresh shrimp, 1.5 lb

Sea salt, .25 tsp

Pepper, .25 tsp

Minced garlic, 3 cloves

Chopped fresh thyme, 1 tbsp

Chopped fresh rosemary, 1 tbsp

EVOO, 3 tbsp – divide

Large orange

1. Zest your whole orange.

2. Add the salt, pepper, garlic, thyme, rosemary, two tablespoons of oil, and the orange zest into a Ziploc baggie. Add in the shrimp, seal, and massage everything together to make sure that the shrimp are coated and everything is combined together. Set to the side.

3. Heat up a large pan, grill pan, or a grill. Coat the cooking surface with the rest of the oil. Place half the shrimp on and cook it for four to six minutes, or until it turns opaque, flip halfway through the cooking time. Place the cooked shrimp in a serving bowl and continue with the rest of the shrimp.

4. As the shrimp is cooking, peel your orange and slice the flesh into bite-size pieces. Add this in with the cooked

shrimp and toss everything together. You can serve now or serve chilled. Enjoy.

Steamed Mussels

Serves: 4

Lemon wedges, for serving

Sea salt, .25 tsp

Pepper, .25 tsp

Lemon slices, 2

Dry white wine, 1 c

Sliced garlic, 3 cloves

Thinly sliced red onion, 1 c

EVOO, 1 tbsp

Small mussels, 2 lbs

1. Place a large colander in a sink and add in the mussels. Clean them with cold water, making sure that the mussels don't sit in standing water. Check to make sure that the shells are all closed. If you find some that aren't, you should discard those, as well as any cracked shells. Leave them in the colander until you need them.

2. Add the oil to a large pan. Cook the onion in the oil for about four minutes, stirring a few times. Mix in the garlic and cook for another minute, constantly stirring. Mix in the salt, pepper, lemon slices, and the wine. Allow this to come up to a simmer and cook for two minutes.

3. Place the mussels in the wine sauce and place on the lid. Cook everything for three minutes, or until the mussels pop open. Shake the pan a few times during the cooking process

4. The shells should all be wide open at this point. Use a slotted spoon to get rid of any mussels that didn't open. Spoon all of the good mussels into a serving bowl and top with the wine sauce. Serve with a couple of lemon wedges if you want.

Cod Stew

Serves: 6

Sliced mushrooms, 3 c

Cod fillets, 1.5 lbs – cut into one-inch pieces

Sea salt, .25 tsp

Pepper, .25 tsp

Dry red wine, .33 c

Sliced olives, 1 c

Chopped roasted red peppers, 12 oz jar

Undrained diced tomatoes, 14.5 oz can

Smoked paprika, .75 tsp

Minced garlic, 2 cloves

Chopped onion, 2 c

EVOO, 2 tbsp

1. Add the oil to a large pot and heat. Cook the onion for about four minutes, stirring a few times. Mix in the smoked paprika and garlic and cook for another minute.

2. Stir in the salt, pepper, wine, olives, roasted peppers, and tomatoes with their juices. Turn the heat up and let everything come to a boil. Mix in the mushrooms and cod and then turn the heat down.

3. Place a lid on the pot and cook for ten minutes. Stir a few times during cooking until the cod flakes easily and is cooked through. Enjoy.

Sicilian Tuna Bowl

Serves: 6

Sea salt, .25 tsp

Pepper, .25 tsp

Rinsed and drained cannellini beans, 15 oz can

Undrained tuna in olive oil, 2 6-oz cans

Sugar, 2 tsp

Crushed red pepper, .25 tsp

Capers, .25 c

Drained sliced olives, .5 c

Minced garlic, 3 cloves

Chopped onion, 1 c

EVOO, 3 tbsp

Chopped kale, 1 lb

1. Fill a large pot with water, about ¾ of the way full, and let it come to a boil. Add in the kale and let it cook for two minutes. This will help to get rid of some of the bitterness in the kale. Drain in a colander and set to the side.

2. Place the empty pot on the stove and add in the oil. Cook the onions for four minutes, stirring occasionally. Mix in the garlic and cook for a minute. Mix in the crushed red pepper, capers, and olives. Cook for a minute, stirring often. Mix in the sugar and the kale. Stir everything until the kale is fully coated in the oil.

Place a lid on the pot and cook for another eight minutes.

3. Set the pot off of the heat and scoop out into a bowl. Stir in the salt, pepper, beans, and tuna. Enjoy.

Zucchini and Tuna Burgers

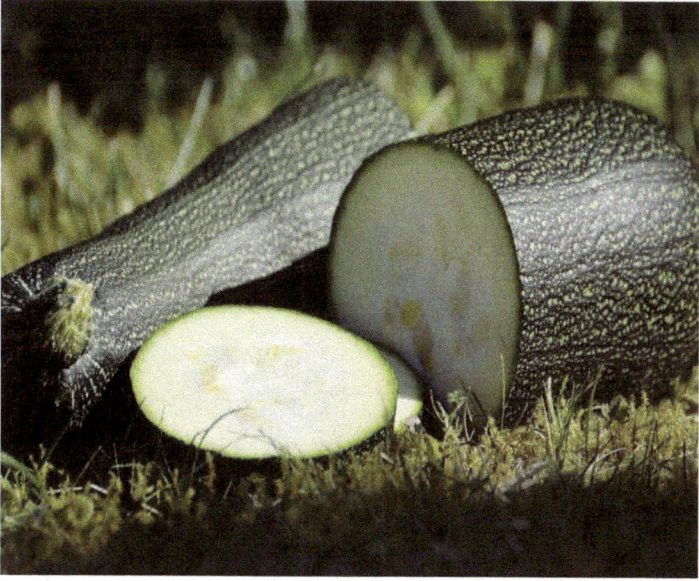

Serves: 4

4 whole-wheat rolls or salad greens, for serving

EVOO, 1 tbsp

Sea salt, .25 tsp

Pepper, .25 tsp

Lemon zest, 1 tsp

Dried oregano, 1 tbsp

Diced red bell pepper, .25 c

Beaten egg

Shredded zucchini, 1 c

Drain tuna, 2 5-oz cans

Toasted whole-wheat sandwich bread, 3 slices

1. Crumble up the toasted bread until you have made about a cup of loosely packed breadcrumbs. Add the crumbs to a bowl and mix in the salt, pepper, lemon zest, oregano, bell pepper, egg, zucchini, and tuna. Use a fork to mix everything and to break up the tuna. Using your hands, form the tuna mixture into four patties that are about a ½ cup size. Lay them on a plate and press down the patties to ¾ inch thickness.

2. Heat the oil in a large pan until it is really hot. This will take about two minutes. Place a patty in the oil and then lower the heat. Let the patty cook for five minutes and then flip and cook for another five minutes. Do this with all of the patties. These can be served on a roll or on top of some salad greens.

Salmon Supper

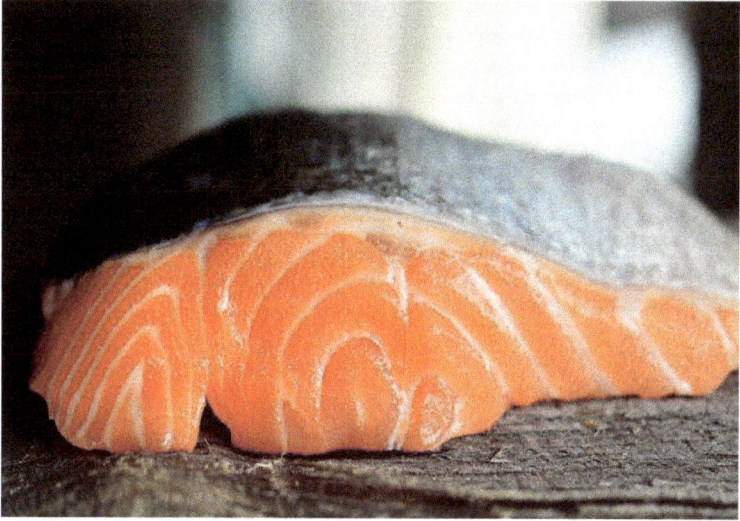

Serves: 4

Lemon juice, 1 tbsp

Skinned salmon fillets, 1 lb cut into 8 fillets

Sea salt, .25 tsp

Pepper, .25 tsp

Water, 1 tbsp

Chopped roasted red peppers, 12 oz jar

Quartered cherry tomatoes, 1 pint

Smoked paprika, 1 tsp

Minced garlic, 2 cloves

EVOO, 1 tbsp

1. Heat the oil in a large pan and add in the smoked paprika and the garlic. Cook this for a minute. Mix in the salt, pepper, water, roasted peppers, and tomatoes. Up the heat, and let everything come to a simmer. Cook this for three minutes, stirring a few times and mashing up the tomatoes with your spoon.

2. Nestle the salmon into the mixture and spoon the sauce over top of the salmon. Place on a lid and let it cook for 10-12 minutes, or until the salmon has cooked all the way through. It should flake easily with a fork.

3. Set the pan off of the heat and add in the lemon juice. Break the salmon up with a fork and stir everything together. Enjoy.

Polenta Fish Sticks

Serves: 4

Cooking spray

Pepper, .25 tsp

Sea salt, .25 tsp

Smoked paprika, .25 tsp

Whole-wheat panko breadcrumbs, .5 c

Yellow cornmeal, .5 c

Skinned fish fillets, 1 lb cut into 20 strips that are ½-inch thick and 1-inch wide (white fish works best)

Milk, 1 tbsp

Beaten eggs, 2

1. Start by placing your oven to 400 and slide a large baking tray in the oven to heat.

2. Mix the milk and eggs together and then carefully coat the fish sticks in the egg wash.

3. Add the pepper, salt, smoked paprika, breadcrumbs, and cornmeal in a large baggie. With tongs, place the egg washed fish sticks and add them to the bag. Make sure you let the excess egg wash drip off first. Seal up the bag and shake until the fish sticks are well coated. You may want to do this just a few at a time.

4. Carefully use oven mitts to take the baking tray out of the oven and spray it with cooking spray. Using your

tongs, lay the fish stick across the hot baking tray. Make sure you leave space between the fish sticks so that they can cook evenly and crisp up.

5. Bake them for five to eight. They should flake easily when done. Enjoy.

Sheet Pan Dinner

Serves: 4

Grape tomatoes, 1 pint

Green beans, 2.5 c

Fish fillets, 4 4-oz fillets – tilapia or cod is best

Balsamic vinegar, 1 tbsp

EVOO, 2 tbsp

Cooking spray

1. Start by placing your oven to 400. Spray two large sheet pans with cooking spray.

2. Mix together the vinegar and oil and set to the side.

3. Lay two fish fillets on each of the sheet pans.

4. Mix together the tomatoes and beans and toss them in the vinegar and oil mixture. Divide the green bean mixture between the two sheet pans, laying them on top of the fish. Flip over the fish fillets, coating them in the oil mixture. Spread everything out evenly on the sheet pans so that everything can cook evenly.

5. Bake these for five to eight minutes, or until the fish is opaque. When the fish starts to flake apart, it is ready to serve.

Grilled Lemon Fish

Serves: 4

Sea salt, .25 tsp

Pepper, .25 tsp

EVOO, 1 tbsp

Medium lemons, 3-4

Cooking spray

Your favorite fish fillets, 4 4-oz fillets

1. Pat the fish fillets dry and let them come to room temperature for ten minutes. Meanwhile, spray your grill with some cooking spray and then heat it up to 400 or med-high. You can also heat up a grill pan on the stove top.

2. Slice a lemon in half, placing one side to the half. Slice this half of lemon along with all of the other whole lemon into ¼-inch thick slices. There should now be about 12-16 lemon slices. Squeeze the juice of the reserved lemon half into a bowl.

3. Mix the oil into the lemon juice and brush them over the fish. Top with some pepper and salt.

4. Lay the lemon slices on your grill or grill pan. Use three to four slices, overlapping them, to make the shape of a fish fillet. Do this for every fish fillet. Lay the fish on the lemon slices and grill them with the lid closed. If you

are cooking them on the stove top, cover them with a lip or some aluminum foil. You don't need to flip the fish unless it is more than a half inch thick.

5. This is cooked through once it starts to flake apart. Enjoy.

Quick Tilapia with Avocado and Onion

Serves: 4

Sliced avocado

Chopped red onion, .25 c

Tilapia, 4 4-oz fillets

Sea salt, .25 tsp

Orange juice, 1 tbsp

EVOO, 1 tbsp

1. Using a 9-inch pie plate, mix together the salt, orange juice, and oil. One fillet at a time, place into the pie plate and coat on all sides with the juice mixture. Once all of them are coated, lay them in the pie dish in a wagon-wheel formation. One end of each fillet should be in the middle of the dish, and the other end will be temporarily draped over the edge. Add a tablespoon of onion to the top of each fish and then fold the end of the fish that is hanging off the end over the onion. There should now be four folded fillets in your pie dish.

2. Cover the dish with some saran wrap, leaving a little section open to allow the steam to vent. Microwave the fish for three minutes. It is cooked when it flakes easily with a fork.

3. Serve the fish topped with some avocado and enjoy.

North African Peanut Stew

Serves: 4

Fresh cilantro, chopped peanuts, pickled hot peppers, for serving

Creamy peanut butter, .33 c

Undrained lentils, 15 oz can

Frozen cauliflower rice, 12 oz package

Undrained diced tomatoes, 28 oz can

Water, .5 c

Sea salt, .25 tsp

Crushed red pepper, .5 tsp

Grated ginger, 1 tsp

Ground allspice, 1 tsp

Cumin, 1.5 tsp

Minced garlic, 3 cloves

Cubed, unpeeled sweet potato

Cubed, unpeeled Yukon Gold potato, 2

Chopped onion, 1 c

EVOO, 2 tbsp

Frozen corn, 1 c

1. Place the corn on the counter to thaw out a little bit as you put the stew together.

2. Add the oil to a large pot and heat. Add in the sweet potato, potatoes, and onion. Cook this for seven

minutes, stirring occasionally. The onion and potatoes should become crispy and golden.

3. Slide the potatoes to one edge and add in the salt, crushed red pepper, ginger, allspice, cumin, and garlic into the empty space. Cook for a minute, stirring constantly. Mix in the water and cook for a minute. Make sure you scrape down the crispy bits from the bottom of the pot.

4. Mix in the tomatoes with juices. Cook everything for 15 minutes. Stir every few minutes, so nothing sticks.

5. As the stew cooks, cook your cauliflower rice following the directions on the package.

6. To the tomato mixture, mixed in the peanut butter, corn, and lentils. Turn the heat down and cook everything for two minutes, or until everything is cooked through. Stir this constantly so that the peanut butter gets mixed in.

7. Serve the stew over top of the cauliflower rice with some cilantro, peanuts, and peppers if you so desire.

Mushroom Bolognese with Polenta

Serves: 4

Sugar, .5 tsp

Whole milk, .5 c

Dry red wine, .5 c

Pepper, .25 tsp

Sea salt, .25 tsp

Nutmeg, .25 tsp

Dried oregano, 1 tbsp

Tomato paste, .25 c

Plain polenta, 18 oz tube cut into 8 slices

Minced garlic, 4 cloves

Finely chopped carrot, .5 c

Finely chopped onion, 1.5 c

EVOO, 3 tbsp – divided

White button mushrooms, 2 8-oz packages

1. Add one of the packages of the mushrooms into your food processor and pulse it around 15 times until chopped up but not pureed. It should look a lot like ground meat. Place the chopped mushrooms to a bowl and repeat the chopping process with the rest of the mushrooms. Set everything to the side.

2. Heat up two tablespoons of the oil in a large pot. Cook the onion and carrot together for about five minutes. Stir everything a couple of times. Mix in the garlic and

mushrooms and cook for another five minutes, stirring often.

3. As your veggies are cooking, add in the rest of the oil to a large pan. Add in four of the polenta slices and cook on each side for three to four minutes or until golden. Take the polenta out and place in a serving dish. Keep this warm by wrapping in foil, and repeat with the other four slices of polenta.

4. In the mushroom mixture, add the pepper, salt, nutmeg, oregano, and tomato paste. Mix everything together and cook for two to three minutes, or until the veggies are soft and have started to brown.

5. Pour in the wine and cook for a couple of minutes, deglazing the bottom of the pot. Cook until most of the wine has evaporated. Turn the heat down.

6. Meanwhile, combine the sugar and milk in a microwaveable bowl and microwave it for 30-45 seconds, or until very hot. Slowly mix the milk into the mushrooms and simmer everything for four minutes, or until the milk has been absorbed. To serve, pour the mushroom mixture over the polenta and enjoy.

Stuffed Tomatoes

Serves: 4

Chopped almonds, .33 c

Honey, 4 tsp

Medium lemon

Sea salt, .25 tsp

Pepper, .25 tsp

Chopped scallions, 2 – green and white parts

Minced fresh mint, .33 c

Minced fresh curly parsley, 1.5 c

Uncooked whole-wheat couscous, .5 c

Water, .5 c

EVOO, 3 tbsp – divided

Beefsteak tomatoes, 8

1. Start by placing your oven to 400.

2. Slice off the top of every tomato and place to the side. Scoop the flesh out and add the seeds, flesh, and tops to a large bowl.

3. Using a tablespoon of the oil, grease a casserole dish. Sit the carved-out tomatoes into the dish and cover everything with foil. Roast the tomatoes for ten minutes.

4. As the tomatoes cook, start making the couscous by boiling a pot of water. Add in the couscous, stir, and set

it off the heat. Place on a lid and let it sit for five minutes. Fluff the couscous with a fork.

5. As the couscous cooks, chop up the tops and flesh of the tomatoes Drain the excess water off of the tomatoes and then measure out a cup of the chopped tomatoes. You can reserve any chopped tomato that is leftover for another use. Place the cup of the tomatoes in a bowl along with the salt, scallions, mint, pepper, and parsley. Stir everything together.

6. Zest the lemon into the bowl with the chopped tomatoes. Cut the lemon in half and squeeze the juice from both halves in. You will want to use a strainer to make sure you don't end up with seeds in the mixture. Mix everything together.

7. Once the couscous is cooked, pour it into the tomato mixture and combine.

8. Carefully take the tomatoes out of the oven and divide the tabbouleh between them. Use a spoon to press down the filling so that you can get as much as possible in them, but make sure you don't press so much that the tomato breaks. Re-cover with foil and cook for eight to ten minutes, or until the tomatoes slightly tender but still a little firm.

9. Before you serve, top each of the tomatoes with a ½ teaspoon of honey and two teaspoons of almonds.

Stuffed Portobello

Serves: 6

Dried oregano, for serving

Shredded mozzarella, 4 oz

Cooking spray

Large Portobello mushrooms, 6 – gills and stems removed

Sea salt, .25 tsp

Crushed red pepper, .25 tsp

Dried oregano, 1 tsp

Chopped tomato, 1 c

Diced zucchini, 2 small

Chopped mushrooms, 3 c

Minced garlic, 2 cloves

Diced onion, 1 c

EVOO, 3 tbsp - divided

1. Add two tablespoons of the oil to a large pan and heat. Cook the onion for about four minutes, stirring a few times. Mix in the garlic and cook for another minute.

2. Mix in the salt, crushed red pepper, oregano, tomato, zucchini, and mushrooms. Cook this for ten minutes, occasionally stirring. Set this off of the heat.

3. As the vegetables cook, heat up a grill pan or a grill to med-high.

4. Brush the rest of the oil over the Portobello caps. Lay the mushrooms stem side down on the grill. Cover and cook them for five minutes. If you are using a grill pan, you can cover them with some foil that has been sprayed with cooking spray.

5. Flip over the caps and add a ½ cup of the vegetables to each cap. Top each mushroom cap with 2 ½ tablespoons of the mozzarella and sprinkle with some extra oregano if you want.

6. Cover, again, and grill for another four to five minutes.

7. Take the Portobellos off of the grill using a spatula and allow them to rest for five minutes before serving.

Eggplant Zucchini Gratin

Serves: 6

Fresh basil, .25 c

Shredded mozzarella, 1 c

Chopped tomato, 1 c

Grated parmesan, .33 c + 2 tbsp – divided

Milk, .75 c

All-purpose flour, 1 tbsp

EVOO, 3 tbsp – divided

Sea salt, .25 tsp

Pepper, .25 tsp

Finely chopped zucchini, 2 large

Finely chopped large eggplant

1. Start by placing your oven to 425.

2. Toss together the salt, zucchini, eggplant, and pepper.

3. Heat a tablespoon of oil in a large pan. Add in half of the vegetables. Stir them a couple of times, then place on a lid and cook them for five minutes. Stir everything a few times while it's cooking. Add the vegetables to a casserole dish.

4. Heat another tablespoon of oil in the pan and add in the rest of the vegetables. Repeat the cooking process with these veggies and then add them to the casserole dish.

5. As the veggies are cooking, heat up the milk for a minute in the microwave and set to the side.

6. Add the flour and the rest of the oil to a medium pot and whisk everything together until blended.

7. Slowly add in the milk, constantly whisking. Continue until the mixture has thickened slightly. Mix in a third of a cup of parmesan, and whisk until melted and combined. Pour this sauce over the veggies and mix everything together.

8. Carefully stir in the mozzarella and tomatoes. Bake for ten minutes, or until the gratin is nearly set and no longer runny. Top with the fresh basil and the rest of the parmesan. Enjoy.

Sweet Potato Burgers

Serves: 4

Whole-wheat rolls, 4 – for serving

Crumbled gorgonzola, .5 c

Sea salt, .25 tsp

Garlic clove

Dried oregano, 1 tbsp

Balsamic vinegar, 1 tbsp

Egg

Old-fashioned rolled oats, 1 c

Chopped onion, 1 c

EVOO, 2 tbsp – divided

Large sweet potato

1. Pierce the potato several times with a fork and microwave it for four to five minutes, or until cooked. Cool slightly then cut it in half.

2. As the potato cooks, heat a tablespoon of oil in a large pan and cook the onion for five minutes. Stir this occasionally.

3. With a spoon, carefully scoop all of the sweet potato flesh out of the skin and place it in a food processor. Add in the salt, garlic, oregano, vinegar, egg, oats, and onion. Process this until smooth. Add in the cheese and pulse it a couple of times to just bring it all together.

Using your hands, form the mixture into four burgers. Flatten the patties to ¾-inch thick.

4. Clean out the pan you used earlier and add in the rest of the oil, heating until very hot. This will take about two minutes. Place the patties into the hot oil and then lower the heat down and cook for five minutes. Flip them and then cook for another five minutes. You can eat these as is, or serve them on whole-wheat rolls.

Lentil Sloppy Joes

Serves: 4

Chopped romaine, 1 c

Chopped seedless cucumber, 1.5 c

Split open whole-wheat pita, 4

Sea salt, .25 tsp

Dried thyme, 1 tsp

Cumin, 1 tsp

Undrained low-sodium diced tomatoes, 14.5 oz can

Rinsed and drained lentils, 15 oz can

Minced garlic, 2 cloves

Chopped bell pepper, 1 c

Chopped onion, 1 c

EVOO, 1 tbsp

1. Heat the oil in a pot and cook the bell pepper and onion for about four minutes. Stir this often. Mix in the garlic and cook for another minute. Mix in the salt, thyme, cumin, tomatoes with their liquid, and lentils. Turn down the heat and cook for ten minutes, or until the majority of the liquid has evaporated. You will need to stir a few times to make sure nothing sticks.

2. Stuff this mixture into each of the pitas. Top with the lettuce and cucumbers.

Pesto Zoodles

Serves: 4

Walnut pieces, .75 c – divided

Packed fresh basil, 1 c

Grated parmesan, 2 tbsp – divided

Sea salt, .25 tsp – divided

Pepper, .25 tsp divided

Crushed red pepper, .5 tsp

Minced garlic, 2 cloves – divided

EVOO, .25 c – divide

Medium zucchini, 4

1. In order to make the zoodles, you will need a spiralizer or a vegetable peeler. Either spiralize your zucchinis or us the peeler to turn the zucchini into long strips.

2. Combine the half the salt, pepper, and garlic, with the crushed red pepper, the zoodles, and a tablespoon of oil. Set to the side.

3. Heat half of a tablespoon of the oil in a large pan. Add in the half of the zoodles and cook them for five minutes, stirring a few times. Add the cooked zoodles to a bowl and repeat this process with the rest of the oil and zoodles. Once cooked, add the zoodles with the rest.

4. As your zoodles cook, make the pesto. With a food processor ass in the rest of the pepper, salt, and garlic, along with ¼ cup of walnuts, the basil leaves, and a tablespoon of parmesan. Flip on the processor and then slowly add in the rest of the oil until the pesto comes together.

5. Pour the pesto over the cooked zoodles and top with the rest of the walnuts and parmesan. Toss everything together and enjoy.

Stuffed Collards

Serves: 4

Grated parmesan, 2 tbsp

Cooked frozen grain medley, 2 10-oz bags

Collard green leaves, 8 – tough stems and tips cut off

Low-sodium crushed tomatoes, 28 oz can

1. Start by placing your oven to 400. Add the tomatoes to a baking sheet and set to the side.

2. Fill up a pot to ¾ full with water and allow this to boil. Add in the collards and cook them for two minutes. Drain. Lay the greens out and pat them dry.

3. To make the collards, place a leaf vertically on the counter and place ½ cup of the grain medley in the middle of the leaf. Fold a long side of the leaf over the filling and then fold over the other long side. They should overlap slightly. Firmly and gently roll the bottom end up until it is slightly square. Carefully place this on the baking sheet with the seam-side down onto the crushed tomatoes. Do this with the rest of the leaves.

4. Top the leaves with the cheese and cover everything with foil. Bake it all for 20 minutes, or until the greens have become tender. Enjoy.

Lamb Stew

Serves: 6

Cooked bulgur or couscous, for serving

Chopped unsalted pistachios, .25 c

Lemon juice, 2 tbsp

Rinsed and drained chickpeas, 15 oz can

Chopped prunes, .5 c

Water, 2 c

Chopped chipotle in adobo sauce, 1 tbsp

Tomato paste, 2 tbsp

Minced garlic, 4 cloves

Sea salt, .25 tsp

Cinnamon, .5 tsp

Cumin, 1 tsp

Diced carrot, .5 c

Chopped onion, 1 c

EVOO, 1 tbsp

Boneless lamb leg steak, 1 lb

1. Slice the meat into inch size cubes and pat them dry.

2. Heat the oil in a large pot and add in the lamb. Cook this for four minutes, stirring just to make sure that the meat browns on every side. With a slotted spoon, set the lamb out on a plate. It won't be completely cooked just yet.

3. Add the salt, cinnamon, cumin, carrot, and onion to the pot and cook for six minutes. Stir everything occasionally. Move the vegetables to the sides of the pot. Place the garlic in the center and cook for a minute, constantly stirring. Add in the chipotle pepper and tomato paste and cook for another minute, stirring constantly and mashing the tomato paste into the veggies.

4. Place the lamb back into the pot with the prunes and water. Turn the heat up to get everything boiling. Lower the heat cook for five to seven minutes, or until the stew has thickened a bit. Mix in the chickpeas and cook for another minute. Take the stew off the heat and mix in the lemon juice. Top with the pistachios and serve with bulgur or couscous if you want.

Marinated Pork Tenderloin

Serves: 6

Chopped mint, 2 tbsp – optional

Tzatziki sauce

Chopped fresh rosemary, 1 tbsp

Greek yogurt, .25 c

Sea salt, .5 tsp

Pepper, .5 tsp

Medium pork tenderloins, 2

Cooking spray

1. Start by setting your oven to 500.

2. Place foil on a sheet pan and place a wire rack on top. Grease with some cooking spray.

3. Lay the pork on the wire rack, folding in the skinny ends of the meat to make sure everything cooks evenly. Rub in some pepper and salt.

4. Stir together the rosemary and yogurt. Using your fingers or a spoon, rub the yogurt mixture over the pork.

5. Place this in the oven to cook for ten minutes. Take the baking sheet out of the oven and flip over the pork

pieces. Roast for another 10-12 minutes or until it reaches at least 145 and the juices run clear. Take the pork off of the rack and onto a cutting board. Allow them to rest for at least five minutes.

6. Slice up the pork and serve it with fresh mint and tzatziki sauce.

Mini Meatloaves

Serves: 6

Pita bread or romaine lettuce, for serving – optional

Olive brine, 2 tbsp

Chopped kalamata olives, .33 c

Greek yogurt, .5 c

Pepper, .25 tsp

Dried oregano, .5 tsp

Egg

Crumbled feta, .5 c

Whole-wheat breadcrumbs, .5 c

Ground beef, 1 lb

Minced garlic clove

Minced onion, .5 c

EVOO, 1 tbsp

Cooking spray

1. Start by placing the oven to 400. Grease a 12-cup muffin tin with cooking spray and set to the side.

2. Heat the oil in a small pan and cook the onion for four minutes. Mix in the garlic and cook for another minute, stirring often. Set this off the heat.

3. Mix the onion mixture with the pepper, oregano, egg, feta, breadcrumbs, and ground beef in a bowl. Use your

hands when you are mixing this together. They work better than a spoon does.

4. Split the mixture into the 12 muffin cups and then bake them for 18-20 minutes, or until it reaches 160.

5. As your meatloaves are baking, mix together the olive brine, olives, and yogurt.

6. Once you are ready to eat, serve the meatloaves on a slice of pita or on a bed of lettuce if you want, top with the yogurt mixture.

Beef Sliders

Serves: 4

Slider whole-grain rolls, for serving – optional

Torn fresh basil, 2 tbsp

Sliced bell peppers, 2

Balsamic vinegar, 1 tbsp

Pepper, .25 tsp

Sea salt, .5 tsp – divided

Minced garlic, 2 cloves

Ground beef, 1 lb

EVOO, 2 tbsp – divided

White button mushrooms, 8 oz package

Cooking spray

1. Place your oven rack to about four inches under the broiler element. Heat your oven to the broil setting.

2. Place some foil on a large sheet pan. Lay a wire rack on the sheet pan and grease it with some cooking spray. Set this to the side.

3. Add half of the mushrooms to a food processor and pulse a few times until they are chopped up and has the appearance of ground meat. Empty into a bowl and repeat with the rest of the mushrooms.

4. Heat a tablespoon of oil in a large pan and add in the chopped mushrooms. Cook for two to three minutes,

stirring often. Once the mushrooms have cooked down and most of the liquid has cooked off, set it off the heat.

5. Mix together the pepper, ¼ teaspoon of salt, garlic, and mushrooms in a bowl. Carefully form this into eight small patties that are about ½-inch thick, and lay them on the prepared rack. You will make two rows of four patties on the sheet pan.

6. Place this in the oven and broil the burgers for four minutes. Flip them over and cook them for three to four more minutes. If all of the burgers aren't getting a lot of action from the broiler, move them around so that the ones who haven't been directly under the broiler are. They should reach 160. Make sure that nothing burns.

7. As the burgers cook, mix together the rest of the salt, vinegar, and the remaining oil. Mix in the basil and the pepper. Stir this gently together just to coat the peppers and basil in the dressing.

8. Once the burgers are cooked, serve them topped with the slaw and on a roll if you so desire.

Tahini Sauce Beef Gyros

Serves: 4

Whole-wheat pita bread, 4 6-inch – warmed

Thinly sliced red onion, 1 c

Lemon juice, 1 tbsp

Greek yogurt, .5 c

Hot water, 1 tbsp – if needed

Peanut butter or tahini, 2 tbsp

Halved green bell pepper

Lamb leg steak, top round, or beef flank steak, 1 lb

Sea salt, .25 tsp

Pepper, .5 tsp

Cumin, 1 tsp

Garlic powder, 1.25 tsp – divided

Dried oregano, 1 tbsp

EVOO, 2 tbsp

Cooking spray

1. Move the top rack of the oven to about four inched under the broiler. Heat your broil up. Place some foil a large sheet pan and top with a wire rack. Grease the rack with cooking spray and set to the side.

2. Mix together the salt, pepper, cumin, a teaspoon of garlic powder, oregano, and oil. Reserve a teaspoon of the mixture and rub the rest into the steak. Lay the steak on the rack. Rub the reserved oil mixture on the

bell pepper and lay it on the rack with the cut-side down. Flatten out the pepper using the heel of your hand.

3. Broil everything for five minutes. Flip the pepper pieces and meat over and broil everything for two to five minutes, or until the pepper has charred and the meat reaches 145. Allow everything to rest for five minutes.

4. As the meat and pepper are cooking, whisk the tahini until it becomes smooth. Add in some hot water if it is sticky. Mix in the rest of the garlic powder, lemon juice, and the yogurt. Whisk until combined.

5. Cut the steak crosswise into quarter-inch strips. Cut the pepper into strips. Divide the onion, bell pepper, and steak between the warmed pita bread. Top with the tahini and enjoy.

Steak and Mushrooms Kebabs

Serves: 4

Sea salt, .25 tsp

Red wine vinegar, 2 tbsp

Pepper, .25 tsp

Medium red onion sliced into 12 wedges

White button mushrooms, 8 oz package

Boneless top sirloin steak, 1 lb

EVOO, 2 tbsp – divided

Rosemary sprigs, 2

Peeled garlic, 4 cloves

Cooking spray

1. Soak 12 ten-inch-long wooden skewers in water. Grease a cold grill with cooking spray and heat to med-high.

2. Slice a section of foil into a ten-inch square. Lay the rosemary and garlic in the center and drizzle in a tablespoon of oil. Wrap this up tightly to make a foil packet. Place on the grill and cover.

3. Slice the steak into 1-inch cubes. Start threading the skewers. Place on a beef cube, mushroom, beef cube, onion wedge, and continue the pattern until you have made all of the kebabs and used up your ingredients. Spray them with the cooking spray and top with some pepper.

4. Cook them on the grill for four to five minutes. Flip, and cook for another four to five minutes. 145 cooks the meat to med-rare, and 160 is medium.

5. Take the foil packet off of the grill, open, and then use tongs to transfer the garlic and rosemary to a bowl. Making sure you don't burn yourself, remove the leaves from the rosemary sprigs. Pour in any juices that accumulated in the packet. Add in the salt, vinegar, and the rest of the oil. Mash up the garlic and stir everything together. Serve this and enjoy.

Spanakopita Pita Pockets

Serves: 4

Whole wheat pita bread, 4 6-inch – sliced in half

Slivered almonds, .25 c

Pepper, .25 tsp

Nutmeg, .5 tsp

Ricotta cheese, .33 c

Crumbled feta, .5 c

Chopped baby spinach, 2 6-oz bags

Minced garlic, 2 cloves

Ground beef, 1 lb

EVOO, 3 tsp – divided

1. Heat a teaspoon of oil in a large pan. Add in the ground beg and cook for ten minutes, breaking it apart as it cooks. Once browned, set it off the heat and drain off the grease. Set to the side.

2. Put the pan back on the heat and in the remaining oil. Add in the garlic, cooking for a minute. Mix in the spinach and cook for two to three minutes, or until it has wilted. Stir everything often.

3. Up the heat and stir in the pepper, nutmeg, ricotta, cook beef and feta. Mix until everything is well incorporated. Stir in the almonds.

4. Place the beef in the eight pita pocket halves and enjoy.

Moroccan Meatballs

Serves: 4

Chopped mint, lemon or orange wedges, and feta cheese, for serving – optional

Low-sodium crushed tomatoes, 28 oz can

EVOO, 1 tsp

Panko breadcrumbs, .33 c

Ground lamb or beef, 1 lb

Egg

Smoked paprika, .25 tsp

Cinnamon, .5 tsp

Cumin, 1 tsp

Chopped raisins, .25 c

Finely chopped onion, .25 c

1. Mix together the egg, paprika, cinnamon, cumin, raisins, and onion. Add in the breadcrumbs and ground beef, using your hands to gently mix everything together. Split the mixture into 20 portions making them as even as possible. Wet your hands slightly and then roll each section into a ball. Clean your hand before continuing.

2. Heat the oil in a large skillet and cook the meatballs for eight minutes. Roll them around every few minutes to help the brown on all sides. They are not going to be cooked through just yet. Place the meatballs on a paper

towel covered plate. Remove the fat from the pan and wipe out with a paper towel.

3. Place the meatballs back in the pan and cover with the tomatoes. Place on a lid and cook until everything starts to bubble. Turn the heat down and let everything cook for seven to eight minutes, or until the meatballs have cooked all the way through. Garnish the meatballs with some fresh citrus, feta, or mint if you want.

Chicken Panzanella

Serves: 6

Honey, 1 tsp

Juice and zest of a lemon

Balsamic vinegar, 1 tbsp

Pepper, .25 tsp

Chopped mint leaves, 3 tbsp

Diced red onion, .25 c

Chopped walnuts, .33 c

Gorgonzola cheese crumbles, .5 c

Halved cherry tomatoes, .5 pint

Halved red seedless grapes, 1 c

Chopped cooked chicken breast, 2 c

EVOO, 5 tbsp – divided

Day-old bread cut into cubes, 3 c

1. Place some foil on a large sheet pan. Place this to the side. Place the rack in the oven at about four inches until the broiler element. Set your oven to broil.

2. Add two tablespoons of oil to the cubed bread and toss everything together with your hands to coat. Spread these across the baking sheet and broil for two minutes. Stir the bread and cook for 30-60 seconds. Keep an eye on the bread so that they become toasted and not burned. Take them out of the oven and set to the side.

3. Mix together the pepper, mint, onion, walnuts, gorgonzola, tomatoes, grapes, and chicken. Add in the bread pieces and carefully mix everything together.

4. Mix together the honey, juice, and zest from the lemon, vinegar, and the remaining oil. Drizzle this over the salad and toss everything together and enjoy.

Chicken Caprese

Serves: 4

Balsamic vinegar, 4 tsp

Torn basil, 2 tbsp

Low-sodium crushed tomatoes, 14.5 oz can

Shredded mozzarella, 1 c

Thinly sliced large tomato

Sea salt, .25 tsp

Pepper, .25 tsp

EVOO, 2 tbsp

Skinless, boneless chicken breasts, 1 lb

Cooking spray

1. Place the rack of the oven about four inches under the broiler. Set your oven to 450. Place some foil on a sheet pan and place a wire rack on the pan and grease the rack with cooking spray. Place it to the side.

2. Slice the chicken into four pieces. Place them in a bag and use a mallet or rolling pin to pound the chicken out so that it is a quarter inch thick. Add in the salt, pepper, and oil. Seal the bag and rub the ingredients into the chicken. Remove the chicken and place it on a wire rack.

3. Let the chicken cook for 15-18 minutes, or until it reaches 165. Switch the oven to broil. Lay the tomato

slices on the chicken and top with some mozzarella. Let the chicken broil for two to three minutes, or until the cheese melts. Make sure that chicken doesn't burn. Take the chicken out.

4. As the chicken cooks, add the tomatoes to a microwavable bowl and microwave for a minute, or until hot. Once you are ready to serve the chicken, place the tomatoes on four plates and top with a chicken breast. Top everything with some balsamic vinegar and basil.

Peach Chicken Legs

Serves: 4

Pepper, .25 tsp

Sea salt, .25 tsp

Smoked paprika, .5 tsp

Garlic, 3 cloves

Cider vinegar, .25 c

Honey, .25 c

Drained sliced peaches, 15 oz can

Cooking spray

Skinless chicken drumsticks, 8

1. Take the chicken out of the refrigerator.

2. Place your oven rack to about four inches under the broiler. Set your oven to 500. Place some foil on a large sheet pan and set a wire rack on top. Grease the rack with some cooking spray and set to the side.

3. Add the pepper, salt, smoked paprika, garlic, vinegar, honey, and peaches in a blender and puree until smooth.

4. Pour this into a pot and let it come up to a boil on med-high. Cook this for two minutes, constantly stirring. Split the sauce between two bowls. You will use the first bowl to coat the chicken. Set the second bowl aside for serving.

5. Brush the chicken with half of the sauce; keep half to give them a second coating. Roast the chicken for ten minutes.

6. Take the chicken out and flip the oven to broil. Brush the rest of the sauce on the chicken and broil for five more minutes. Flip the chicken oven and cook for another three to five minutes. It should reach 165, or until the juices run clear. Serve the chicken legs with the reserved sauce.

Artichokes and Lemon Chicken

Serves: 4

Skin-on bone-in chicken thighs, 4 6-oz thighs

Large artichokes, 2

Sea salt, .5 tsp

EVOO, 3 tbsp – divided

Large lemons, 2

1. Set your oven to 450 and place a large sheet pan in the oven and let it heat up. Tear off four sheets of foil that are about eight by ten. Set this aside.

2. Zest a lemon into a large bowl. Slice both lemons in half and squeeze all of their juices into the bowl. Mix in two tablespoons of oil and the salt. Set to the side.

3. Rinse the artichokes under cool water and dry them. With a sharp knife. Slice 1 ½ inches off of the tip of each of the artichokes. Cut a quarter inch off of the stem. Plunge the artichoke in the lemon juice mixture so that they don't turn brown. Coat them on all sides. Place one artichoke, flat-side down, in the middle of each of the foil packets. Wrap them up tightly. Place these to the side.

4. Coat the chicken in the remaining lemon mixture.

5. Carefully take the sheet pan out of the oven and pour on the rest of the oil. Tilt the pan to spread it around. Carefully place the chicken, with the skin-side down, on the hot pan. Place the artichoke packets on the pan.

6. Roast everything for 20 minutes, or until it reaches 165. The juices should run clear. To check and make sure that the artichokes are done, pull on a leaf. If the leaf removes easily, it's done. Serve the chicken and artichokes together.

Chicken Rice Bowls

Serves: 4

Fresh mint leaves, for serving

Sesame seeds, 4 tsp

Chopped seedless cucumber, 2 c

Chopped dried apricots, .5 c

Chopped cooked chicken breast, 2 c

Sea salt, .25 tsp

Cinnamon, .75 tsp

Cumin, 1 tsp

Water, 1 tbsp

Lemon juice, 1 tbsp

Chopped scallions, 2 tbsp – white and green parts

Greek yogurt, .25 c

Tahini, .25 c

Uncooked instant brown rice, 1 c

1. Follow the package directions to cook the brown rice.

2. As the rice cooks, combine the salt, cinnamon, cumin, water, lemon juice, scallions, yogurt, and tahini. Split the mixture in half. Mix the chicken into one of the bowls of the sauce.

3. Once the rice is cooked, stir it into the second bowl of the tahini mixture.

4. To make the bowls, split the chicken mixture into four bowls and spoon in the rice to each bowl. Next, to the chicken, add the apricots, and in the last section, add the cucumber. Top with mint and sesame seeds if you want.

Chicken and Potatoes

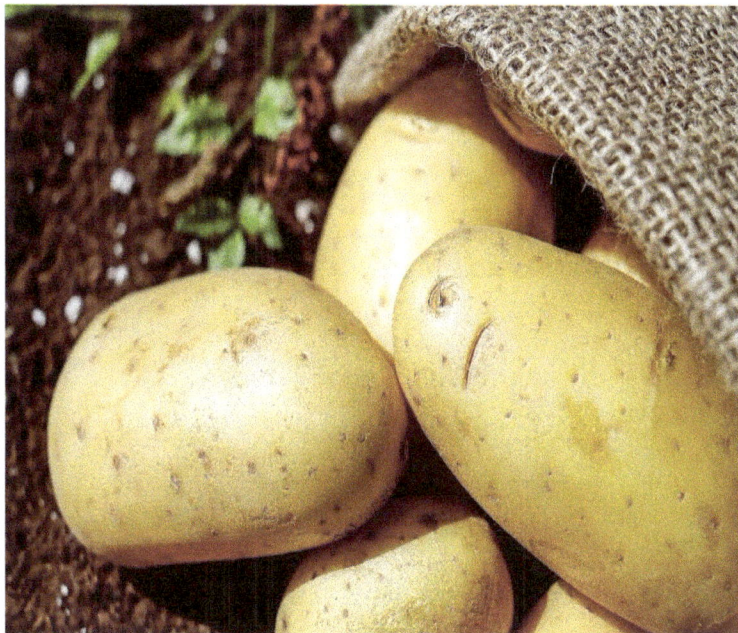

Serves: 6

Lemon juice, 1 tbsp

Chopped flat-leaf parsley, 1 c

Pepper, .25 tsp

Sea salt, .25 tsp

Dijon mustard, 1 tbsp

Low-sodium chicken broth, 1 c

Dry white wine, .25 c

Minced garlic, 2 cloves

Cubed, unpeeled Yukon Gold potatoes, 1.5 lb

EVOO, 1 tbsp

Skinless, boneless chicken thighs, 1.5 lb - cubed

1. Dry off the chicken and heat the oil in a large pan. Add in the chicken and cook for five minutes. Stir the chicken to make sure that it browns on all sides. Take the chicken out of the pan using a slotted spoon and set in a plate. It is not going to be completely cooked yet.

2. Add the potatoes to the skillet and cook them for five minutes. Stir them to make sure that they become crispy and golden on all sides. Push the potatoes to the side. Add in the garlic and cook for a minute. Pour in the wine and cook until nearly evaporated. Add in the chicken pieces, pepper, salt, mustard, and chicken broth. Up the heat and let everything boil.

3. Once it has started to boil, place a lid on the skillet and turn down the heat. Cook for 10-12 minutes, or until the potatoes become tender and the chicken is cooked through.

4. In the last minutes of the cooking process, mix in the parsley. Take the pan off the heat and mix in the lemon juice. Enjoy.

Almond Crusted Chicken

Serves: 4

Almonds, 1 c

Skinless, boneless chicken breast tenders, 1 lb

Pepper, .25 tsp

Sea salt, .25 tsp

Dijon mustard, 1 tbsp

Honey, 1 tbsp

Cooking spray

1. Start by placing your oven to 425. Place parchment on a sheet pan and top with a wire rack. Grease with cooking spray.

2. Mix together the pepper, salt, mustard, and honey and then add in the chicken. Gently toss everything together so that it is coated. Place to the side.

3. With a food processor, chop up the almonds, making them about the size of sunflower seeds. Dump the nuts out onto the sheet of parchment and spread out. Press the chicken tenders into the nuts so that they are coated. Lay the chicken on the rack

4. Bake the chicken for 15-20 minutes or until the juices run clear and reaches 165.

5. Serve and enjoy.

Shrimp and Feta

Servings 4

Cubed feta, 8 oz

Peeled, deveined shrimp, 1 lb

Cubed tomatoes, 2

Olive oil, 4 tbsp

Chopped garlic, 2 cloves

Sliced green pepper, 1

Sliced onion, 1

1. Place a skillet on medium and warm the olive oil. Add in the onion, garlic, and green pepper. Cook for five minutes.

2. Add in the tomatoes, stir well and simmer 15 minutes.

3. Add in the feta and shrimp. Season with pepper and salt.

4. Cook an additional 15 minutes.

5. Taste and adjust seasonings if needed.

Spicy Salmon

Servings 4

Salt, .5 tsp

Salmon steaks, 4

Juice of one lemon

EVOO, 2 tbsp

Crushed red pepper flakes, 1 tsp

Minced garlic, 4 cloves

1. Take the garlic and salt and mash together to make a paste.

2. Add in lemon juice, red pepper flakes, and EVOO, keep mashing until you have a smooth mixture.

3. Place mixture on top of salmon and place in the refrigerator for two hours.

4. You need to warm your oven to 450.

5. Take the salmon out of the refrigerator for 20 minutes. Place onto a greased baking sheet.

6. Place into the oven and bake 20 minutes.

Baked Cod

Servings 1

Pepper to taste

Salt to taste

Parchment paper cut 20 inches

Cod, 4 oz

Olive oil, .5 tbsp

Juice of .5 lemon

Pitted olives, 5

Halved, cherry tomatoes, 5

Sliced potatoes, 2

1. You need to warm your oven to 350.

2. Take the parchment paper and place the sliced potatoes on top.

3. Place the lemon juice, olives, and tomatoes into a bowl and stir to combine.

4. Place the fish on top of the potatoes and pour the tomato mixture on top of fish.

5. Fold the parchment into a small package to seal the edges.

6. Place on a baking sheet and put into the oven for 20 minutes.

Roasted Fish with Potatoes

Servings 4

Skinless salmon fillets, 4

Cubed new potatoes, 12

Dill, .25 tsp

Grated orange zest, .5 tsp

White vinegar, 3 tbsp

EVOO, 3 tbsp

Orange juice, 3 tbsp

1. You need to warm your oven to 420. Line a baking sheet with parchment paper.

2. Place the orange juice, EVOO, white vinegar, orange zest, and dill. Stir well to combine.

3. Use two tablespoons of this mixture and coat the potatoes. Place on the prepared baking sheet.

4. Put into the oven and cook for 20 minutes.

5. Take the remaining mixture and put on the salmon fillets.

6. When the potatoes have cooked for 20 minutes, take out of the oven and place the salmon fillets on top of the potatoes.

7. Place back into the oven for another 15 minutes.

Skillet Shrimp

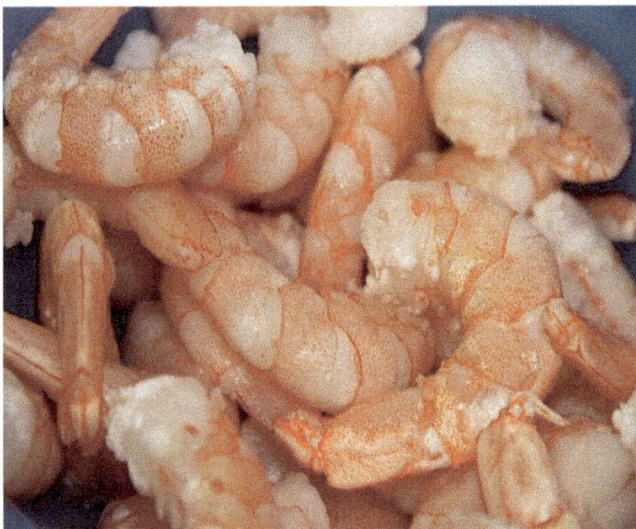

Servings 4

Pepper

Salt

Sliced onion, 1

Thyme, 1 tsp

Minced garlic, 2 cloves

EVOO, 2 tbsp

Peeled, deveined shrimp, 1 lb

1. Preheat your broiler.

2. Place a skillet on medium heat and warm the EVOO.

3. Add the onion and garlic to the skillet and cook for three minutes.

4. Add the pepper, salt, thyme, and shrimp.

5. Place the skillet under the broiler for six minutes.

Snacks

Lemony Hummus

Serves: 6

Lemon juice, 3 tbsp – reserve the liquid

Drained chickpeas, 15 oz can

Whole-grain crackers or raw veggies, for serving – optional

Sea salt, .25 tsp – optional

Garlic, 2 cloves

EVOO, 3 tbsp – divided

Peanut butter, 2 tbsp

1. Add the chickpeas and two tablespoons of the reserved liquid to a food processor, along with the garlic, peanut butter, lemon juice, and two tablespoons of oil. Mix everything together for a minute. Scrape down the sides and mix for another minute, or until it becomes smooth.

2. Place the hummus in a bowl and drizzle the top with the rest of the oil. You can add a sprinkling of salt if you want and serve with your favorite veggies sticks or crackers.

Mano'ushe Flatbread

Serves: 6

Sea salt, .25 tsp

EVOO, 3 tbsp

Sesame seeds, 3 tbsp

Dried thyme, 3 tbsp

Cooking spray

Package of whole-wheat pizza dough, 16 oz

1. Start by placing your oven to 450. Grease a cooking tray with cooking spray.

2. Split the dough out into three equal size balls. Lightly flouring a counter, roll out the dough balls into a six-inch circle. Lay the dough circles onto your prepared cooking tray.

3. Mix together the salt, oil, sesame seeds, and thyme. Using a brush or spoon, brush the herbed oil onto the dough circles until you have used it all up.

4. Bake the dough for ten minutes, or until the edges begin to brown and crisp up and the oil has cooked through the dough. If you don't want to fool with pizza dough, you can just use pre-made pita. If doing so, only cook them for five minutes.

5. Take the flatbreads out of the oven and slice each circle in half. Enjoy.

Crunchy Chickpeas

Serves: 4

Zest of ½ orange

Sea salt, pinch

Dried thyme, .25 tsp

EVOO, 2 tsp

Rinsed and drained chickpeas, 15 oz can

1. Start by setting your oven to 450.

2. Lay the chickpeas out on a hand towel and rub them carefully until they are dry.

3. Lay the chickpeas out on a baking tray. Drizzle on the oil and then top them with salt and thyme. Zest half of an orange over the top of the chickpeas and then mix everything together with your hands.

4. Bake these for about ten minutes. Once the first ten minutes are up, carefully reach into the oven, using a mitt, and shake the baking tray a bit to move the chickpeas around. You should not take the tray out of the oven. Bake them for another ten minutes. Carefully taste them to see if they are crunchy enough for you. You can cook them for about three more minutes if they are not crunchy enough or browned. Enjoy.

Energy Bites

Serves: 6

Rolled oats, .25 c – quick or old-fashioned

Chopped pecans, .5 c

Diced dried figs, .75 c

Honey, 2 tbsp

Peanut butter, 2 tbsp

Ground flaxseed, 2 tbsp

1. Combine the peanut butter, flaxseed, oats, pecans, and figs. Drizzle in the honey and mix it all together. Using a wooden spoon tends to work the best because you can really press all of the ingredients together. Once everything is mixed together, freeze the dough for five minutes so that you can handle it better. The peanut butter makes it a bit sticky.

2. Split the down into four sections. Wet your hands slightly with water. This is the tricky part if you get your hands too wet, they will stick and too dry they will stick. You will have to play around with it a little bit.

3. Using your hands, form each of the four sections into three bites. This should make a total of 12 energy bites.

4. You can enjoy these right away, or you can freeze them for a few minutes to help them firm up before enjoying. They will last refrigerated for a week.

Honey Almonds

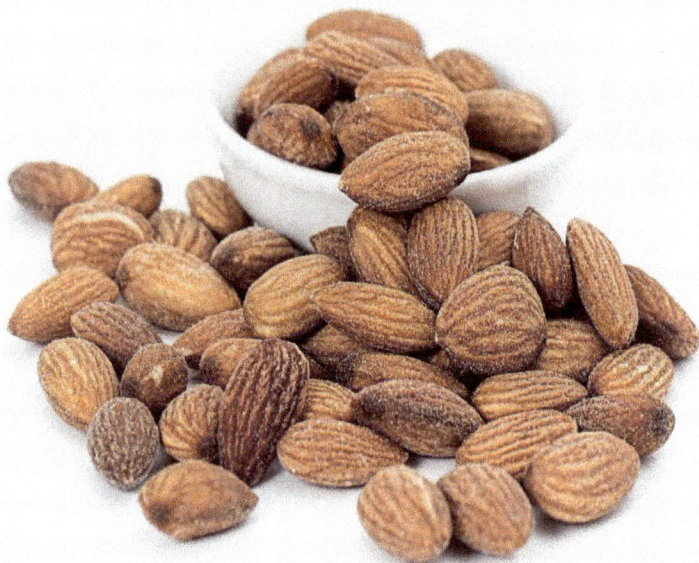

Serves: 6

Cooking spray

Honey, 1 tbsp

Sea salt, .25 tsp

Minced fresh rosemary, 1 tbsp

Whole, raw, shelled almonds, 1 c

1. Add the salt, rosemary, and almonds to a large pan and cook them for a minute. Stir everything frequently.

2. Add in the honey and cook for three to four minutes, stirring often, until the almonds are completely covered and are beginning to darken around the edges.

3. Take them off the heat and spread the almonds out on a greased cooking tray. Let the almonds cool for ten minutes. Break them up and enjoy.

Eggplant Relish

Serves: 6

Chopped olives, .5 c

Red wine vinegar, .5 c

Chopped tomatoes 1.5 c

Chopped roasted red peppers, 12 oz jar

Sea salt, .25 tsp

Globe eggplants cut into ½-inch cubes

Minced garlic clove

Finely chopped onion, 1 c

EVOO, 2 tbsp

1. Add the oil to a large pan and heat.

2. Add in the onion to cook for about four minutes, stirring a few times. Mix in the garlic and cook for a minute. Up the heat and mix in the salt and eggplant. Cook this for five minutes, stirring occasionally.

3. Mix in the vinegar, tomatoes, and peppers. Place a lid on the pan and cook everything for ten minutes. Make sure you stir it a few times so that it doesn't burn or stick. If it appears to be sticking and burning, lower the heat and add in a tablespoon of water.

4. Set this off the heat and stir in the olives. Allow this to rest for a few minutes so that the liquid can absorb. Stir

this again and enjoy. You can also pour it into a jar and keep it in the fridge for ten days. It tends to taste better if you let it sit for a day so that the flavors have time to marry.

Romesco Dip

Serves: 10

Garlic, 2 cloves

Dry-roasted almonds, .5 c

Undrained diced tomatoes, 14.5 oz can

Drained roasted red peppers, 12 oz jar

Assortment of sliced raw vegetables

Torn day-old bread, .66 c

EVOO, .25 c

Pepper, .25 tsp

Sea salt, .25 tsp

Smoked paprika, 1 tsp

Red wine vinegar, 2 tsp

1. Add the pepper, salt, smoked paprika, vinegar, garlic, almonds, tomatoes with juices, and roasted peppers to a food processor or blender.

2. Start to puree the ingredients together on medium. Carefully add the oil in as the processor is running. Continue to mix until the dip is smooth and combined.

3. Add in the bread and puree everything together.

4. Serve the dip with the slices of raw vegetables. You can also store it in a lidded jar. It should keep for a week.

Cheese and Fruit Board

Serves: 4

Cubed cheese, 1 c – Asiago, Manchego, feta, Gorgonzola, or goat

Jarred, canned, or cured vegetables, 1 c – artichoke hearts or roasted peppers

Sliced raw vegetables, 2 c – cherry tomatoes, cauliflower, broccoli, celery, or carrots

Finger fruits, 2 c – figs, grapes, cherries, or berries

Sliced fruits, 2 c – peaches, plums, pears, or apples

1. Clean off all of your produce and slice the ones that need to be.

2. Place the fruits and veggies on a wooden board or tray. You can add on some spoons for the berries and knife or fork for the cheeses. Serve with napkins and plates.

Papas Tapas

Servings 6

Sea salt, .5 tsp

Pepper, .25 tsp

EVOO, 2 tsp

Sliced Yukon gold potatoes, 3

Toppings of choice

1. You need to warm your oven to 400.

2. Sprinkle the sliced potatoes with pepper and salt. Drizzle with olive oil. Place in the oven for ten minutes. Turn potatoes over and cook another ten minutes.

3. Top each slice with your favorite Bruschetta toppings or toppings of choice.

Blue Cheese Figs

Servings 2

Honey, 1.5 tsp

Chopped rosemary, 1 sprig

Blue cheese, 2 tbsp

Figs, 3

1. Slice the figs in half.

2. Spread each half with some blue cheese and top with rosemary.

3. Drizzle with honey and enjoy.

Parmesan Walnuts

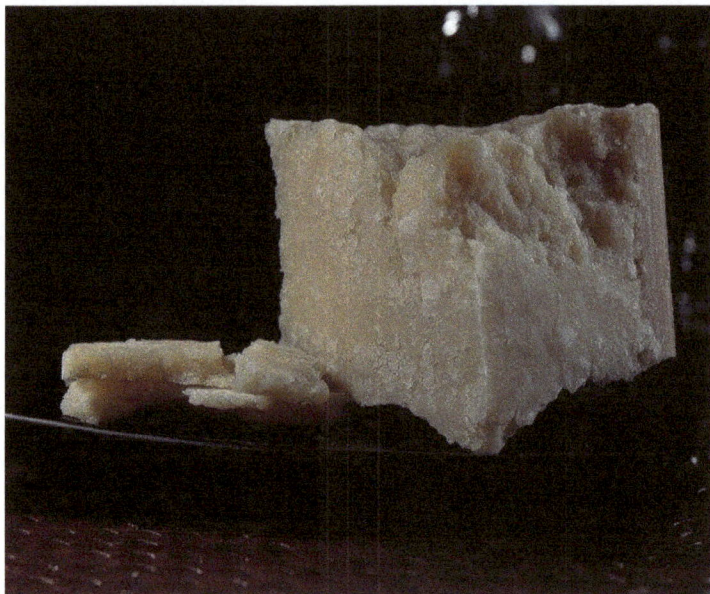

Servings 8

Cayenne pepper to taste

Egg white, 1

Walnuts, 2 c

Garlic salt, .5 tsp

Parsley flakes, 1 tsp

Italian seasoning, .5 tsp

Grated Parmesan cheese, .5 tsp

1. You need to warm your oven to 250.

2. Lightly grease a baking sheet with olive oil.

3. Place all ingredients except walnuts and egg whites into a bowl.

4. Whisk the egg white and add in walnuts. Stir well to coat.

5. Add coated walnuts to cheese mixture. Stir well to coat.

6. Pour onto a greased baking sheet and bake for 30 minutes.

7. These can be eaten either warm or cold.

Blueberry Avocado Bang

Servings 2

Maple syrup to taste

Berries of choice, 2 c

Avocados, 2

Cubed, frozen banana, 1

1. Place all ingredients into a blender except maple syrup. Blend until smooth. Add more ice or water if needed.

2. Pour into glasses and drizzle on some syrup.

Peanut Butter Popcorn

Servings 4

Wildflower honey, .25 c

Agave syrup, .25 c

Peanut butter, .33 c

Chopped peanuts, .33 c

Sea salt, .5 tsp

Popcorn kernels, .5 c

Peanut oil, 2 tbsp

1. Place the peanut oil and popcorn into a pot and sit to coat.

2. Place the pot on medium. Once the kernels begin to pop, gently shake the pot until all the kernels have popped.

3. In another saucepan, add agave and honey. Cook on low for five minutes. Add in the peanut butter and stir until peanut butter has melted.

4. Pour peanut butter mixture over popped popcorn and toss to coat. Enjoy.

Desserts

Honey Walnut Brownies

Serves: 9

Pitted and stemmed cherries, 9

Chopped walnuts, .33 c

Salt, .25 tsp

Baking powder, .25 tsp

Unsweetened dark chocolate cocoa powder, .33 c

Whole-wheat pastry flour, .5 c

Greek yogurt, .5 c

Vanilla, 1 tsp

Eggs, 2

EVOO, .25 c

Honey, .33 c

Sugar, .5 c

Cooking spray

1. Start by setting your oven to 375 and place that rack at the middle point of your oven. Grease a square baking dish with cooking spray.

2. Using either a stand mixer or a hand mixer, beat together the oil, honey, and sugar and creamy. Slowly mix in the vanilla and eggs. Lastly, beat in the yogurt until you have a smooth better.

3. Whisk together the salt, baking powder, cocoa powder, and flour together. Pour the flour mixture into the honey mixture and beat everything together until well incorporated. Stir in the walnuts.

4. Pour the batter into your baking dish. Press the cherries into the tops of the brownies, evenly spacing them so that you have three rows of three. This will mean when you cut the brownies; a cherry will be in the center of each one.

5. Cook your brownies for 18-20 minutes, or until completely set. Take them out of the oven and let them cool on a rack for about five minutes. Slice into nine squares and enjoy.

Orange Rice Pudding

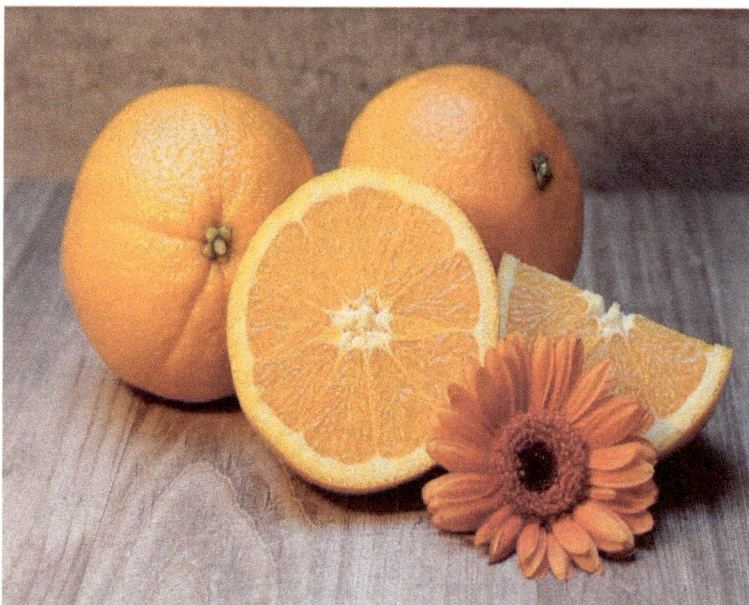

Serves: 6

Vanilla, 1 tsp

Cinnamon, .5 tsp

Honey, .25 c

Uncooked instant brown rice, 1 c

Orange juice, 1 c

Milk, 2 c

Beaten eggs, 2

Sea salt, pinch

EVOO, 2 tsp

Medium orange, 2

Cooking spray

1. Start by setting your oven to 450. Great a large sheet pan with cooking spray and set to the side.

2. Slice the oranges, unpeeled, into ¼-inch thick rounds. Brush them with some oil and sprinkle the tops with salt. Lay the orange slices on the sheet pan and cook them for four minutes. Flip them over and cook for another four, or until they start to brown. Take them out of the oven and place to the side.

3. Working close to the stove, crack the eggs into a bowl. In a pot, combine the cinnamon, honey, rice, orange juice, and milk. Let this come up to a boil, stirring all the time. Lower the heat down and let this simmer for ten minutes, stirring often.

4. With a measuring cup, remove ½ cup of the rice mixture and beat it into the eggs. As you are constantly stirring the rice mixture, pour the tempered eggs into the pot. This will keep your eggs from scrambling. Cook the rice mixture on low for a couple of minutes, or until thickened. You need to stir constantly and make sure that it does not boil. Set it off the heat and mix in the vanilla.

5. Allow the pudding to sit for a few minutes so that the rice will soften. The rice will still be a little bit chewy, but it will be cooked through. If you want your rice to be softer, you can let it sit for half an hour. Serve the pudding at room temp or warm with a roast orange on top.

Lemon Fool

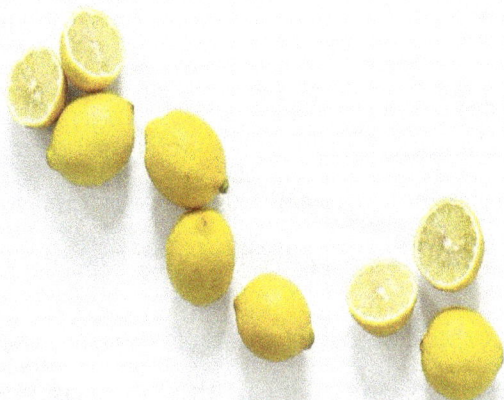

Serves: 4

Fresh mint leaves and fruit, for serving

Heavy cream, .66 c

Honey, 3.5 tbsp – divided

Cornstarch, 1.5 tsp

Cold water, .25 c

Medium lemon

Greek yogurt, 1 c

1. Place the beaters from your mixer and large glass bowl in the refrigerator to chill. Place the yogurt in another glass bowl and lay this in the fridge to chill as well.

2. Using a zester or a Microplane, zest your lemon into a microwavable safe bowl. Cut the lemon in half and squeeze the juice into the bowl. Mix in the cornstarch and water. Stir in three tablespoons of the honey and then microwave the mixture for a minute, stir, and then heat again in 15-second intervals until it has become thick and is bubbling. Be careful not to burn yourself on the mixture.

3. Take the bowl of yogurt out of the fridge and beat in the warm lemon mixture. Slide this back into the refrigerator.

4. Take the large bowl and beaters out of the fridge. Put your mixer together using the chilled beaters and add the cream to the cold bowl. Beat the cream until it

forms soft peaks. This will take about a minute to three minutes, depending on how fresh your cream is.

5. Remove the chilled yogurt mixture from the fridge and carefully fold this into the whipped cream with a rubber spatula. When you do this, lift and turn the mixture so that you don't cause the cream to deflate. Chill this for at least 15 minutes, but no longer than an hour before serving.

6. To serve, spoon into four dessert dishes and top with the remaining honey. If you want, you can serve it with some mint and fresh fruit.

Dark Chocolate Pomegranate Bark

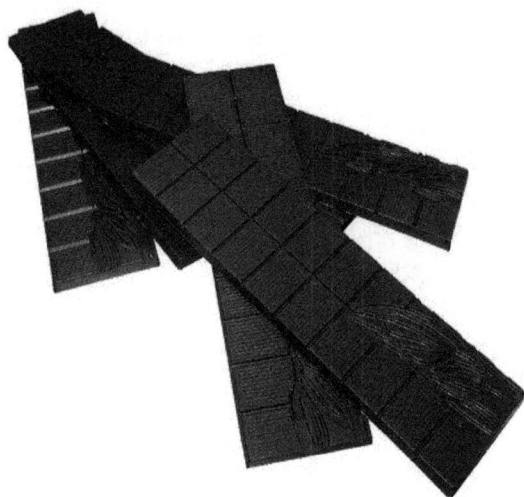

Serves: 6

Fresh pomegranate seeds, .5 c

Dark chocolate chips, 1 c – or – dark chocolate, 8 oz

Sea salt, .5 tsp

Uncooked quinoa, .5 c

Cooking spray

1. Using a medium-sized pot, grease it well with cooking spray and heat. Add the quinoa and toast it for two to three minutes, stirring often. Make sure that the quinoa does not burn. Take the pot off of the stove and stir in the salt. Remove two tablespoons of the quinoa to use later for the topping.

2. Break up your chocolate into big pieces and place them in a gallon-size bag. With a meat mallet, pound the chocolate into some pieces. If using chocolate chips, you can skip this part and just add the chocolate to a microwavable bowl. With your chocolate in the bowl, microwave for a minute and then stir until it melts completely. If you need to you can heat it for 10 seconds more, and stir until it melts. Mix in the toasted quinoa.

3. Place some parchment on a baking sheet and pour the chocolate mixture on the sheet and spread it out evenly across the pan. Sprinkle on the quinoa that you held

back and then top with the pomegranate seeds. Press everything into the chocolate using the back of a spoon.

4. Freeze this for 10-15 minutes, or until firm. Take this out of the freezer and break it into about two-inch size pieces. Keep in a bag in the fridge until you are ready to enjoy.

Whipped Ricotta with Stone Fruit

Serves: 4

Mint, 4 sprigs for garnish

Freshly grated nutmeg, .25 tsp

Whole-milk ricotta, .75 c

EVOO, 2 tsp

Nectarines or peaches halved and pitted, 4 – or plums or apricots, 8

1. Grease a cold grill pan or grill with cooking spray. Heat up to medium.

2. Chill a large bowl in the refrigerator.

3. Brush the halved fruit with some oil. Lay the fruit, cut-side down onto your heated grill and cook them for three to five minutes or until they form grill marks. If you are using a grill pan, you will probably have to do this in two batches. Flip the fruit over with tongs. Cover the grill, or cover them with foil if using a grill pan, and cook them for four to six minutes. You should be able to easily pierce the fruit with a sharp knife. Place to the side to cool.

4. Take the chilled bowl out of the fridge and add in the ricotta. With an electric mixer, beat the ricotta for two minutes on high. Beat in the nutmeg and honey for a

minute. Divide the grilled fruit between four bowls and top with the whipped ricotta and a sprig of mint.

Yogurt Affogato

Serves: 4

Vanilla Greek yogurt, 24 oz

Dark chocolate chips, 4 tbsp

Chopped unsalted pistachios, 4 tbsp

Hot espresso, 4 shot – or – strong brewed coffee, .75 c

Sugar, 2 tsp

1. Divide the yogurt between four bowls or tall glasses.

2. Stir half of a teaspoon of sugar into each of the espresso shots, or mix all of the sugar into the coffee.

3. Divide the coffee or the espresso between the four glasses of yogurt.

4. Top each with a tablespoon of chocolate chips and pistachios. Enjoy.

Dark Chocolate Fruit Kebab

Serves: 6

Dark chocolate, 8 oz

Blueberries, 24

Seedless grapes, 24

Pitted cherries, 12

Hulled strawberries, 12

1. Place some parchment on a sheet pan. Lay out six 12-inch wooden skewers.

2. Thread your fruit onto the skewers in this pattern: strawberry, cherry, two grapes, two blueberries, strawberry, cherry, two grapes, and two blueberries. Repeat with the rest of the fruits and skewers. Lay them on your sheet pan.

3. Heat the chocolate in a microwavable safe bowl for a minute. Stir until the chocolate has completely melted.

4. Place the chocolate in a small plastic bag and twist it all to the corner of the bag and snip off the corner. Drizzle the chocolate over the fruit kebabs.

5. Place the sheet pan in the freezer and chill for 20 minutes and enjoy.

Date Truffles

Servings 10

Cocoa powder, .5 c

Cinnamon, 1 tsp

Orange zest, .75 tsp

Shredded coconut, .5 c

Chopped pecans, 1 c

Brewed coffee, 12 oz

Chopped dates, 3 c

1. Put the dates into the warm coffee and let them sit for five minutes.

2. Take the dates out of the coffee and mash until smooth.

3. Add in the cinnamon, orange zest, coconut, and pecans. Stir well to combine.

4. Using your hand make balls out of this mixture. You might have to dip your hands into the water if the mixture begins to stick to your hands.

5. Place the cocoa powder onto a shallow plate. Once you have formed the mixture into balls, roll in cocoa powder to coat.

Chocolate Mousse

Servings 6

Zest of one orange

Salt

Sugar, .5 c

Eggs, 7

Orange liqueur, 3 tbsp

EVOO, .66 c

Melted dark chocolate, 9.5 oz

1. Separate the eggs into two different bowls. The whites go in one bowl, the yolks into another.

2. Place the melted chocolate into a bowl with the orange liqueur and olive oil. Mix well.

3. Whisk the egg yolks with half of the sugar until well combines. Add this to the chocolate mixture and whisk until smooth.

4. Add in the salt and the rest of the sugar. Continue to whisk until everything is incorporated.

5. Pour mixture into small dessert bowls and put into the refrigerator for 20 minutes before serving.

Strawberry Banana Smoothie

Servings 2

Ice, .25 c

Flaxseed oil, 1 tbsp

Skim milk, 1.25 c

Fat-free yogurt, 1.25 c

Orange juice, 2 tbsp

Banana, 1

Sliced strawberries, .75 c

Rolled oats, 4 tbsp

1. Place all the ingredients into a blender and process until completely smooth and creamy.

Summer Granita

Servings 4

Raspberries, .5 c

Lemon juice, 2 tbsp

Orange juice, .25 c

Water, .5 c

Sugar, .5 c

Diced nectarines, 1 lb

1. Place the nectarines into a pot. Add sugar and stir. Place the pot on medium heat and bring to a boil. Let boil for ten minutes.

2. Add in the raspberries and give everything a good stir.

3. Add in the juices and more sugar if needed. Stir well.

4. Place into a freezer safe container and put into the freezer for 30 minutes.

5. After 30 minutes are up, use a fork and stir until it forms granules. Spoon into bowls and enjoy.

Porcupines

Servings 36

Salt, .5 tsp

Vanilla, 1 tsp

Flour, .75 c

Eggs, 2

Shredded coconut, 1 c

Chopped walnuts, 1 c

Chopped dates, 1 c

EVOO, 1 tbsp

1. You need to warm your oven to 350. Place a piece of parchment paper onto a baking sheet.

2. Put the olive oil, vanilla, and eggs into a bowl and whisk until well combined.

3. Add in dates and walnuts and stir to combine.

4. Add in flour and salt. Keep mixing until everything is well incorporated.

5. Using a spoon and your hand, make balls until all the mixture is gone. Place the coconut onto a shallow plate. Roll the balls in the coconut until well coated.

6. Place on prepared baking sheet and bake 15 minutes.

Getting Started

When anybody begins anything new, they want immediate results. They want to achieve their goals fast and without having to do much. Having these expectations can cause disappointment and frustration, and this makes them conclude that this lifestyle isn't for them. This is the biggest reason why most people stop their diets. First off, you have to believe you are going to succeed and make an effort to improve your health. Second, you need to make changes gradually, and they will soon become new habits.

Eating like the people from the Mediterranean region can promote health benefits and decrease the risk of developing chronic diseases. Following a Mediterranean eating pattern can decrease certain forms of cancer, reduce cardiovascular disease, manage blood pressure, decrease risks of type 2 diabetes, improve eye health, and protects against cognitive decline. It is better than a low-fat diet to help you lose weight. Following the Mediterranean diet isn't just healthy, it is satisfying and delicious. Foods that were once thought about as being unhealthy or high in fats, like whole grains, olives, olive oil, and nuts will soon become a part of your daily life. This new lifestyle lets you eat all the fresh vegetables and fruits you like. The best thing about this diet is you don't have to do any major changes to what you should already be eating. There are a few tweaks you will need to do to make sure you incorporate everything you need to so you will be successful in your new lifestyle.

The following steps can help you eat the Mediterranean way daily:

1. Be active

Following the Mediterranean lifestyle encourages you to eat healthy foods but you also have to exercise. When you are home, you could play with your children, clean the yard or house, walk the dog, ride a bike, go roller skating, take the stairs rather than using the elevator. If you need to go to the store, park further from the building, if at all possible. It might make your trip a bit longer, but you will begin to notice changes to your body.

2. Eat meals with family

Plan to eat dinner at home with your family no less than two times a week. You will have fun and also bring yourself some health benefits. Stop picking up fast food on the way home. Get the children involved and spend time cooking homemade, healthy meals. This gives you the chance to be creative and surprise your family with tasty new foods.

Don't eat while sitting in front of the television. Slow down while sitting at the table with friends and family. Savor what you eat. You will enjoy your food and company more. When you eat slowly, it allows you to tune in to your fullness signals and your body's hunger.

3. Change butter to healthy oils

Start using extra virgin olive oil instead of margarine or butter. Olive oil is a great source of monounsaturated fats. Mixing extra virgin olive oil with some balsamic vinegar is great to dip bread in, and it is healthier than butter. If a recipe includes unhealthy fats, replace the same amount with olive oil. This is great for your heart, and the dish will taste even better. Eating olive oil and staying away from saturated fats, mayonnaise, and butter is the main purposes of this diet. Olive oil can be used for marinades, dressings, and cooking. Try to eat four tablespoons each day as long as it stays in your calorie budget.

4. Stay away from salt

Spices and herbs are full of antioxidants. These can raise the nutrient values of meals and lessen the level of sodium. It has been found that salt can increase blood pressure. You could use sea salt.

5. Have a snack of seeds or nuts

Have a handful of sunflower seeds, walnuts, or almonds instead of reaching for cookies, chips or any other processed foods that are usually loaded with trans fats, saturated fat, and sugars. Low-fat, calcium-rich foods or nonfat plain Greek yogurt with some fresh fruit added in are portable and healthy snacks. You can eat about three ounces of seeds or nuts each week as long as it stays within your caloric budget. Stay away from heavily salted, honey-roasted, and candied seeds and nuts.

6. Eat fish rather than red meat

For most Americans, it is hard to eat fish twice a week and stay away from red meat. Make sure you don't fry your fish. It needs to be baked or grilled. This component of the Mediterranean diet is of great importance due to its anti-inflammatory properties. Fatty fish such as tuna, sardines, salmon, or herring are great replacements for meat.
You can eat while meat poultry like chicken or turkey breast. Limit intake of red meat to once or twice a month and choose lean cuts of meat. Eliminate or limit all processed meats.

7. Rethink sweets

You need to limit your sugar intake. Eat less than three servings each week of high sugar drinks and foods like beverages, desserts, candies, or sugar-sweetened snacks.
If you want dessert, pick a fruit. Don't grab a bag of chips, grab a piece of fruit.
Fruits are a great source of antioxidants, vitamin C, and fiber. Fresh fruit is a great way to indulge your sweet tooth. If it helps you to eat more, add some brown sugar or honey on your grapefruit or pears. Keep fresh fruit on your counter or in a desk drawer, so you have a healthy snack at hand.

8. Eat legumes

Legumes are a huge component of this diet. They are a great substitute for meat. Beans are high in antioxidants and minerals. They are a huge source of fiber and protein, so they can help you lose weight in the long run.

9. Use whole grains instead of refined flour

Consume whole grain products rather than foods such as white rice and white bread. Try out some millet, barley, oatmeal, brown rice, popcorn, or quinoa. A bowl of oatmeal is great for breakfast. Barley is filling because it is full of fiber; pair it with some mushrooms for a wonderful soup. Quinoa is a great substitute for white bread or potatoes. These foods are great for a healthy breakfast and have nutritional value. Check the label and make sure the first ingredient listed is whole wheat when picking any grain-based foods like pasta and bread.

10. Consume alcohol in moderation

It is normal for people from the Mediterranean region to drink red wine with meals. Don't drink alcohol at any other times and never to excess. People who drink red wine in moderation have less heart disease than people who completely abstain. Red wine can raise good HDL cholesterol. It can thin the blood and makes it clot less. It contains antioxidants that keep your arteries from holding on to LDL cholesterol which causes plaque buildup. Just remember that one drink is equal to five ounces of wine.

11. Consume seasonal produce

Try to shop at your local farmer's market to find fresh produce. Try to eat three to eight servings of vegetables daily. A serving size is between one half and two cups. It all depends on what vegetable you are eating. Pick various colors and try to eat the rainbow. Consuming a variety of colors will give you more vitamins and antioxidants. Consume more dark leafy greens like turnip greens, chard, spinach, kale, and collards. Put vegetables in the center of your plate instead of on the side.

Eat two cups of fruits daily. Include berries as often as possible. Make eating a ritual and never eat while on the computer or watching television. Begin your day with a cheddar and spinach omelet.

Conclusion

Thank for making it through to the end of *Mediterranean Diet for Beginners*, let's hope it was informative and able to provide you with all of the tools you need to achieve your goals whatever they may be.

You have learned everything you need to know about the Mediterranean diet and this way of life. You can easily start this diet today. In fact, I'm sure you will. It's an easy diet to sustain. There are no foods that are explicit "can't have." You can enjoy lots of delicious foods without feeling like you are on a diet. Take what you have learned and live a healthier life.

Book 2

Alkaline Diet

The Complete Guide for Beginners.
Eat well with Alkaline Diet
Cookbook.

Delicious Alkaline Recipes

Introduction

Have you been looking for information on the alkaline diet and how it affects the body, but you've yet to find the straightforward information that you want? People who believe in the diet say that replacing acidic foods with alkaline foods will improve your health, fight off diseases, and help you lose weight. However, what about the evidence behind these claims?

Without sounding too technical, the body is constantly working to maintain a healthy pH balance. It likes it when it's a little on the basic or alkaline side. In the following chapters, we will look at what pH is and how it works, but as of right now, the important thing to know is that the scale runs from 0 to 14. Anything over 7 is alkaline and below 7 is acidic.

The Standard American Diet is full of foods that produce acid. It's full of fatty and fried foods, dairy products, red meat, alcohol, refined sugar, and processed carbs. This diet does a lot to the body and very little of it is good. It messes with the liver, kidneys, and the digestive system. This can end up causing health problems like cancer, hypertension, and renal disease.

Nevertheless, if you start filling up your plate with alkaline foods, such as vegetables, beans, leafy greens, fruits, sprouted grains, and more, you will be giving your body a bunch of healthy nutrients and vitamins. Healthy foods will make your cells healthy. A large number of recipes in this book will ensure that you are always satisfied and never bored.

When you get started with the book, you may find that it all seems overwhelming. Don't worry, it is really rather simple. Eating an alkaline diet means that you will choose whole foods and plant-based foods over unhealthy processed foods. There is no need to count calories or remove entire food groups. All you need to do is make sure that you consume more alkaline forming foods than acidic forming foods. You'll be surprised at how quickly you learn what foods you should and shouldn't eat.

The alkaline diet is also perfect for everybody. Also, while it may not have been designed with weight loss in mind, it will help you lose weight. The foods that you do eat will leave you feeling full as well.

It's also a good idea to make sure that you keep up with a regular exercise program, get plenty of sleep, hydrate, and practice some stress-reducing activities.

There are lots of books on this subject on the market, thanks once more for selecting this one! Every effort was created to make sure it's stuffed with the maximum amount of helpful data as attainable, please enjoy!

The Alkaline Diet

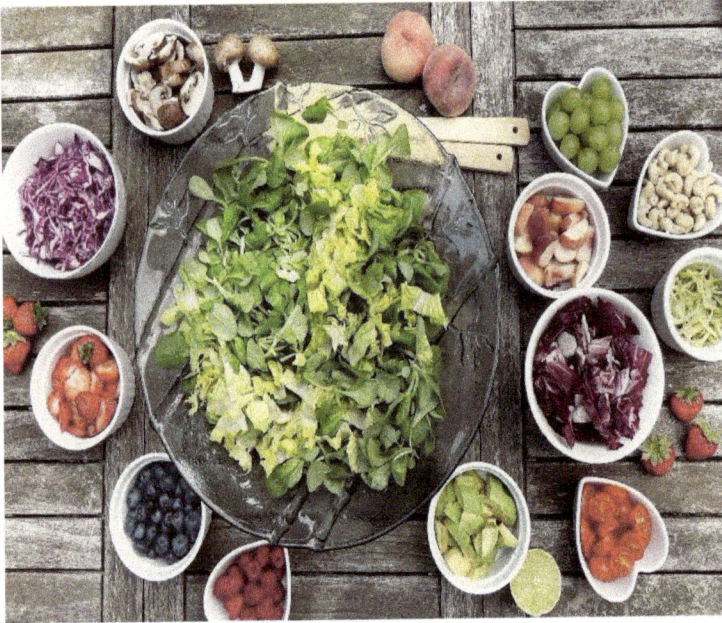

The main principle behind the diet is a philosophy that believes the foods we eat can easily alter the chemistry of our bodies. It all depends on if the food is alkaline or acidic. Basically, our body's pH will change depending on what foods we eat.

You need to understand that when our bodies need energy, it begins to burn food. This process is very controlled and takes place in an environment that our bodies control. When our bodies break down the foods we consume and get the energy from them, we are burning the foods but in a very controlled, slow way. This is what is known as your metabolism, the conversion of food into energy. This works a lot like a fire because it involves a chemical reaction to break down the food. These chemical reactions happen in a controlled and slow manner.

It is just like when you burn wood in your furnace when we burn foods, they are going to produce waste that is sometimes called "ash". This waste product could be either alkaline or acid.

These "ashes" are what alters the pH in our body. It all depends on the mineral, sulfur, or protein content in the food. Consuming foods that leave behind acidic ash like refined carbs, processed foods, fried foods, or sugar can, with time, increase inflammation and this leaves us vulnerable to disease. The bottom line is that if our bodies get exposed to huge amounts of acidic "ash", it will slowly begin to get more vulnerable to diseases because the immune system is getting weaker.

Our bodies house many organs that are very good at eliminating and neutralizing acid. There is a limit to the amount of acid our bodies can handle effectively. The Alkaline Diet doesn't try to change the pH in the blood but removes the stress of trying to maintain a healthy pH in the body by giving it the tools to thrive. Foods that form alkaline like plant proteins, tubers, vegetables, and whole fruits are all alkaline since they are anti-inflammatory, natural, fresh foods that are delicious and rich in antioxidants, chlorophyll, minerals, and vitamins. On the other hand, when our bloodstream gets impacted by a large level of alkalinity, it forms a protective layer that will try to keep our bodies healthy.

This diet is more of an eating plan rather than a diet. It is used to improve our health. Since it has an emphasis on fresh fruits and vegetables, its basis is on the idea that after the foods we eat get absorbed and digested, they will reach the kidneys as eight base- or acid-forming compounds.

There have been many techniques used to look at foods and figure out their base or acid load on the body. Some foods are going to be more base- or acid-producing than others. Surprisingly cheddar is more acid forming than egg whites. Spinach is more base-forming that watermelon.

It is thought that a diet that is high in foods that are acidic will disrupt the blood's pH level and then will trigger the loss of minerals like calcium while the body tries to restore its natural equilibrium. This imbalance is what causes us to be susceptible to illnesses.

The alkaline diet doesn't just help improve your health, it can slow the aging process, preserve muscle mass, and protect against many other health problems such as osteoporosis, kidney stones, cardiovascular disease, diabetes, and the common cold. This diet can also help you lose weight and boost your energy levels.

For these reasons, it is recommended that we try to choose foods that are high in alkalinity.

The following categorizes the various types of foods based on their "ashes".

- Alkaline: Foods like fruits, nuts, legumes, and vegetables.

- Neutral: Foods that contain starches, fats, and sugars

- Acidic: Foods like alcohol, eggs, grains, dairy, poultry, fish, and meats

Here is a bit of background about the alkalinity/acid of a normal diet and points about how this diet can help the human body:

- Researchers think that there has been a huge change from the hunger/gatherer civilization to what we have today. With the agricultural revolution and the mass industrialization of the foods we eat in the past 200 years, the foods we eat have a lot less chloride, magnesium, and potassium. It does have a lot more sodium as compared to other diets.

- Our kidneys keep the electrolyte levels normal. When the kidneys get exposed to very acidic substances, the electrolytes have to be used to fight acidity.

- The ratio of sodium and potassium in normal diets today has changed drastically. Potassium should outnumber sodium by ten to one but the ration has dwindled down to one to three. When eating a "normal" American diet, we now eat three times more sodium than potassium in an average day.

- These changes to our diets have caused an increase in metabolic acidosis. Basically this means the pH levels in our bodies aren't optimal anymore. Besides that, most people suffer from problems like magnesium and potassium deficiency.

- This causes the aging process to accelerate, degenerates bone and tissue mass, and the gradual loss in the functioning of organs. Because of the high degree of acid in our bodies it forces our bodies to get the minerals it needs from our tissues, organs, cells, and bones.

What is pH?

Let's begin with a little refresher in chemistry class and remind ourselves about what pH is. A simple definition is how much hydrogen ion concentration there is in our body. The initials pH is short of "power of hydrogen". The "p" stands for "potent" or the German word for power and "H" stands for the element symbol for hydrogen. The pH scale ranges from one to 14. Seven is neutral. A pH of less than seven will be acidic. Solutions that have a pH of more than seven are alkaline. In order for us to have good health, our bodies need to be a little bit alkaline. Our blood's pH and other cellular fluids should be around a pH of 7.365 to 7.45. It is important to realize that pH levels will vary a lot throughout the body. Some parts will be acidic while others will be alkaline. Basically, there isn't a set level. Our stomachs are loaded with hydrochloric acid and this gives it a pH of between 2 to 3.5. This makes it very acidic. It needs to be this acidic so it can break down the foods that we consume and kills harmful bacteria. Our saliva ranges from pH levels of 6.8 to 7.3. The skin has a pH level of 4 to 6.5. This acts as a protective barrier from the environment. Our urine has a pH that will vary from alkaline to acid. It all depends on what your body needs in order to balance our internal environment due to the foods we eat.

The measurement that is most important will be your blood's pH. It needs to keep in a very narrow range between 7.365 to 7.45. This might seem simple but instead of our pH operating within a mathematical scale, it operates within a logarithmic scale in multiples of ten. This means that it will take ten times the amount of alkalinity to be able to neutralize an acid. If there is a jump from six to seven, it might not seem like much but it will take ten times the amount of alkalinity to neutralize this amount. Basically, a pH of five will be 100 times more acidic than a pH of seven. A pH of four will be 1,000 times more acidic. Does this help you understand?

Don't begin stressing about staying in or falling out of that range. Remember our bodies are pretty great at regulating the pH of your blood. Our bodies don't "find" the balance. It has many parts that do this and keeps the blood's pH between 7.365 and 7.45 at all times. If you make poor lifestyle and diet choices, your body works harder to keep the balance. If you want to address the inflammation and acidity in your body by changing your dietary choices to foods that are more alkaline, it will help balance your system and bring your body back to its best vitality.

Even the smallest of alterations to the pH level of different organisms can cause massive problems. Because of the environmental concerns like increasing the deposition of CO_2 in the ocean, its pH level has dropped from 8.2 to 8.1 and the many different life forms that live in the ocean have suffered a lot. The pH level is critical for plant growth and it can affect the mineral content of foods we consume. The human body, soil, and minerals in the ocean are buffers that help maintain the optimal pH level. When there is a rise in acidity, minerals will fall.

- Blood pH

You know that the body is constantly working to make sure that you maintain healthy pH levels in your body. The tricky thing is, there are three liquids in the body that are typically at slightly different pH levels. Overall, they are mostly controlled by the same things. The first thing we are going to look at is blood pH.

Are normal pH range for your blood is 7.35 to 7.45. This means that the blood is normally naturally alkaline or basic. When compared to stomach acid, which is around 3 to 5.5, you can see the big difference. The stomach is supposed to be at this acidic level to break down the foods that you eat. Ironically, if stomach acid becomes more acidic or more basic, it can create the same symptoms of acid reflux, but that's a different discussion. This low pH helps you to digest food and destroys the germs that may enter your stomach.

What can cause the pH of your blood to change or hit levels that are abnormal?

Health problems are typically the most common cause of the blood become too alkaline or acidic. Also, a change in normal blood pH levels can signal a medical emergency or health condition. This can include:

- Poisoning

- Drug overdose

- Hemorrhage

- Shock

- Infection

- Gout

- Lung disease

- Kidney disease

- Heart disease

- Diabetes

- Asthma

Acidosis refers to when your blood pH level drops to anything below 7.35 and starts to become too acidic. Alkalosis refers to when your blood pH level increases to more than 7.45 and starts to become too alkaline. There are two main organs that work hard to help keep your blood pH levels normal:

- Kidneys – These organs work by remove the acid through your urine so that you excrete it.

- Lungs – These organs work by getting rid of carbon dioxide through your breathing.

The different forms of blood alkalosis and acidosis depend greatly on the reason for it. The top two causes are:

- Metabolic – These types of problems most often occur when your blood pH changes due to an issue of condition within the kidneys.

- Respiratory – These types of problems most often occur when your blood pH changes due to a breathing or lung condition.

It is normal for the blood pH levels to be tested as part of a blood gas test. This type of test is also sometimes referred to as an ABG test, or arterial blood gas test. It works by measuring how much carbon dioxide and oxygen is in your blood. Your general practitioner may choose to test your blood pH as a normal part of your year health screenings, or if you already suffer from certain health conditions. Blood pH tests do require having blood removed using a needle. The lab will be sent the blood sample, and perform the test.

There are at-home blood pH tests when you can do by pricking your finger. These tests won't provide you as accurate of a reading as a test at your doctor's office will. Using a urine pH litmus paper test will not provide you with your blood's pH level, but it can let you know if there is something that isn't right.

Let's take a moment to look more closely at some reasons why your blood pH levels my move out of the normal range.

High blood pH, also known as alkalosis, will happen if the pH of your blood rises above the normal range. There are many different causes for the high blood pH levels. You may have a temporary increase in your blood pH with simple illnesses. There are some foods that can also cause your blood to become more alkaline. There are also more serious causes to this alkalosis that can create further problems.

First off is fluid loss. Losing too much water can cause your blood pH levels to increase. This is due to the fact that you also lose some blood electrolytes, which are minerals and salts, when you lose water. These include potassium and sodium. Diarrhea, vomiting, and sweating can cause excess fluid loss. Medications and diuretic drugs can also cause a person to urinate more often, leading to higher blood pH levels. Treatment for fluid loss requires you to make sure you are getting plenty of fluids and making sure you electrolytes are replaced. Some sport drinks can you accomplish this. Your doctor may also look at your medications and stop any that may be causing the fluid loss.

Next, kidney problems can cause high blood pH levels. Your kidneys play a large role in keeping your blood pH normal. A kidney problem can then cause an accumulation of alkalinity in your blood. This is due to the fact that the kidneys won't remove any excess alkaline substances through your urine. For example, the kidneys could improperly filter bicarbonate back into the blood. There are medications and other treatments that can help to lower your blood pH levels.

When there is blood acidosis, it can affect the way every organ in your body functions. Low blood pH is more common issue than high blood pH. Acidosis is often a warning sign to some health problem that is not being controlled.

There are some health conditions that can cause natural acids to build up within the blood. Some forms of acids that can end of lowering blood pH include:

- Carbonic acid

- Hydrochloric acid

- Phosphoric acid

- Sulphuric acid

- Keto acids

- Lactic acid

An improper diet can cause problems. Eating a diet that is imbalanced can create a temporary low blood pH level. Not eating enough or going for extended periods of time without eating can create more acid in the blood. Try to avoid eating too many acid-forming foods, which include:

- Grains – rice, pasta, bread, and flour

- Fish

- Meat

- Eggs

- Poultry – turkey and chicken

- Dairy – yogurt, cheese, and cow's milk

You balance your blood pH by eating more alkaline-forming foods. These most often include dried, frozen, and fresh fruit, and fresh and cooked veggies. Stay far away from fad diets or starvation diets. When trying to lose weight, do so in a healthy, safe way following a balanced diet.

Another cause for low pH levels in the blood is due to diabetic ketoacidosis. If you suffer from diabetes, you blood can end up becoming acidic if you don't properly regular your blood sugar levels. Diabetic ketoacidosis occurs when the body is unable to make enough insulin or use it properly.

Insulin helps by moving sugar from the foods that we eat into the cells of the body. This is where the body will then burn it as fuel. If insulin is unable to be used, you body starts to break down the stored fat in your body to power itself. This releases an acid wasted known as ketones. If the body is not able to regulate this process, the acid will build up and trigger low blood pH.

It is important that you seek out emergency care if your blood sugar level is over 300 milligrams per deciliter. If you suffer from any of the following symptoms, speak with your doctor:

- Confusion

- Stomach pain

- Fruity-smelling breath

- Shortness of breath

- Vomiting or nausea

- Weakness or fatigue

- Frequent urination

- Excess thirst

Diabetic ketoacidosis is most often a sign that diabetes is not being treated properly and is out of control. This can sometimes be the first signs of diabetes for some. Making sure your diabetes is well treated will help keep your blood pH balanced. It may require a strict diet and exercise plan, insulin injections, and medications in order to stay healthy.

A third cause of low blood pH is metabolic acidosis. This is when low blood pH is caused by kidney disease or failure. This occurs when the kidneys are unable to remove acids from your body through urination. This will increase the acids in your body and lower your blood pH.

The most common symptoms of metabolic acidosis are:

- Heavy breathing

- Fast heartbeat

- Headache pain

- Vomiting and nausea

- Loss of appetite

- Weakness and fatigue

Treatment for this problem will often include medications to help the kidneys work better. In more serious cases, it may require a kidney transplant or dialysis. Dialysis works by cleaning the blood.

The last cause of low blood pH is respiratory acidosis. When the lungs aren't functioning probably to remove carbon dioxide quickly from the body, the blood pH levels will lower. This will most often happen if a person suffers from a chronic or serious lung condition, such as:

- Diaphragm disorders

- Chronic obstructive pulmonary disease

- Pneumonia

- Bronchitis

- Sleep apnea

- Asthma

People who are obese, have had surgery, or who abuse opioid painkillers or sedatives are at a higher risk of developing respiratory acidosis. In some cases, the kidneys are able to pick up the slack and remove the excess blood acids through excretion. A person may need to be given extra oxygen and medications like steroids and bronchodilators to help the lungs function properly. In really serious cases, mechanical ventilation and intubation may have to be used in those with respiratory acidosis in order to bring the blood pH back to normal.

- Urine pH

The next type of pH we are going to look at is urine pH. Urine is made up of waste products, salts, and water that are excreted through the kidneys. The balance of these different compounds can affect the acidity level of the urine.

According to the American Association for Clinical Chemistry, the average pH of urine is 6.0, but it can range from 4.5 to 8.0. Any levels under 5.0 is considered acidic urine, and any levels above 8.0 is considered basic urine.

Sometimes different laboratories will have different ranges as to what they consider to be normal pH levels for the urine. One of the main things that affects the pH of your urine is the things that you eat. If you go to the doctor, they will often ask what foods you have eaten before they evaluate the results of a urine pH test.

If, before a test, you have eaten more acid-form foods, you urine is going to be more acidic. The same goes for having eaten more alkaline foods. If a person has extremely high pH levels in their urine, which means it is more alkaline, it could be a sign of some medical conditions, like:

- Urinary tract infections

- Kidney stones

- Other kidney-related disorders

A person can also have high urine pH levels if they have experienced prolonged vomiting. Vomiting causes the body to get rid of stomach acid, which causes of the bodily fluids to become more basic.

When urine is acidic, it creates an environment conducive for kidney stones, as well. When the urine is acidic, it can also be a sign of several severe medical conditions, like:

- Starvation

- Diarrhea

- Diabetic ketoacidosis

As you will notice, much of this is the same of the pH levels of the blood. There are also certain medications that can affect the pH of the urine. Sometimes doctors will have a patient withhold certain medications the day or night before they are going to have a urinalysis.

- Saliva pH

The last pH we are going to look at is saliva pH. The normal pH range for saliva is 6.2 to 7.6. The things you drink and eat can change the pH of your saliva. For example, the bacteria in the mouth breaks down the carbohydrates that you eat, which releases aspartic acid, butyric acid, and lactic acid. This will lower your saliva pH levels. Age also plays a big role in this. Adults will often have more acidic saliva pH levels than children do.

Just like every other area of your body, your mouth needs to keep a balanced pH. Your saliva pH levels can drop to lower than 5.5 when you have been drinking a lot of acidic beverages. When this occurs, the acids in your mouth will begin to break down your tooth enamel.

If your tooth enamel becomes too thin, your dentin will then be exposed. This can end up causing discomfort when you consume sugar, cold, or hot beverages. Just to give you an example of foods and drinks that can do this, here are some numbers:

- Cherries have a pH of 4

- American cheese has a pH of 5

- White wine has a pH of 4

- Soft drinks have a pH of 3

It's easy to spot unbalanced saliva pH levels. Some of the most common indicators are:

- Tooth cavities

- Sensitivity to cold or hot beverages or food

- Persistent bad breath

If you want, you can even test the pH of your saliva. In order to test the pH of your saliva, you will need to find some pH strips. These can easily be found online or in drugstores. Once you have your strips, this is what you do:

- Make sure you don't eat or drink anything for at least two hours before testing.

- Allow your mouth to fill with saliva and then swallow this or spit it out.

- Allow your mouth to fill with saliva again and then place a small amount on one of your pH strips.

- The strip will then react to your saliva. It will change colors based on how alkaline or acidic your saliva is. The container that your pH strips came should show you a color chart. Place your strip next to the chart to match up the colors and find out what your saliva's pH level is.

In order to make sure that you saliva pH stays balanced it's important that you eat foods that are in a healthy pH range. It's also important that you don't let yourself be deprived of important vitamins and minerals. There are some more efficient ways to make sure that your saliva pH remains balanced.

- Stay away from sugary soft drinks. If you must drink them, try to drink them quickly and chase them with some water. Sipping sugary drinks over a long period of time does more damage.

- Limit your black coffee. Adding in some creamy, non-sugary, can help to cut the acidity of the coffee.

- Avoid brushing your teeth immediately after consuming high-acidic drinks like beer, wine, cider, fruit juices, or soft drinks. These types of drinks will soften up your tooth enamel. If you brush too soon after consuming these things, you will further damage your enamel.

- Chew some sugar less gum after you have consumed any beverages or food. Chewing gum will cause your mouth to produce more saliva and it will help to bring your pH level back to normal. It is also believed that xylitol can prevent bacteria from sticking to your tooth enamel.

- Keep yourself hydrated so make sure you drink plenty of water.

Harmful Effects of an Imbalanced pH

You should know how important it is to maintain a balanced pH. This section will tell you about the fatal consequences of changes to the pH. If the pH level in the body gets too alkaline, a symptom called Alkalosis is going to happen. When the body is put under these conditions, you will begin to experience a loss of electrolytes, liver disease, lower oxygen levels, etc. Here are some symptoms of alkalosis:

- Tingling in the face

- Problems breathing

- Seizure

- Sudden onset of muscle spasms

- Twitching

- Light-headedness

- Confusion

On the other hand, if the body starts to get too acidic, your body will enter into a state of acidosis. There are some risks to acidosis like:

- Lethargy

- Breathlessness

- Fatigue

- Confusion

- Kidney damage

- Insulin resistance

- Diabetes

- Increased risk of heart disease

- Renal complications

- Lactic imbalance

- Respiratory problems

- Metabolic problems

Acidosis can be brought on by a diet that isn't balanced and that contains a lot of animal products with only a few vegetables and fruits. Here are some symptoms of acidosis:

- Vomiting

- Nausea

- Increased heart rate

- Arrhythmia

- Diarrhea

- Muscle weakness

- Seizures

- Coughing

- Shortness of breath

- Confusion

- Sleepiness

- Headache

- Loss of consciousness

- Coma

The Alkaline Lifestyle

Studies have been shown that when acidosis is induced and caused by the diet, it is an actual phenomenon. It needs to be recognized and treated, it can be treated by changes to the diet and has significant relevance.

Here are some conditions that the Alkaline Diet could help prevent:

- Heart disease, stroke, and hypertension

A diet high in acidic foods has been associated with higher mortality rates. Researchers studied over 44,000 men and 36,000 women in a 15 year time span. With both women and men, they showed higher mortality rates in the ones who ate a high acid-based diet as compared to ones who ate a diet rich in fresh vegetable and fruits.

Another study in 2016 found that people who had high PRAL had an increase in developing atherosclerotic cardiovascular disease and were put into a high risk group as compared to people who had lower PRAL scores.

Around 33% of adults are diagnosed with high blood pressure. This condition will increase the danger for stroke and cardiovascular disease. There are several risk factors for cardiopathy and high blood pressure, as well as being overweight and inactive. There are very distinct and clear links between the risks and the foods you eat. A normal American diet is known to be high in animal products and very low in vegetables and fruits. It can cause low urine pH and metabolic acidosis. High dietary acid could cause hypertension and could increase the risk of heart disease. Basically, the alkaline diet is high in magnesium and potassium that promotes healthy blood pressure. Consuming more alkalizing foods could shift the number of minerals in your body and could decrease the risk of heart disease.

- Kidney stones

One in ten people will have problems with kidney stones in their lifetime. There are several risk factors involved but a diet that is high in sugar, sodium, and protein could increase the risk by adding more nutrients that promote stones than the kidneys will be able to filter. This is very true in diets that are high in sodium that will increase how much calcium your kidneys have to filter. Foods that promote stones include uric acid that is found in animal proteins, phosphorus, sodium, oxalate that is found in chocolate and some nuts, and calcium. These can all contribute to a low-grade metabolic acidosis. Healthy, young people can filter these foods, when we begin aging, we will experience a decline in kidney function. Passing kidney stones isn't a picnic and new research shows that dietary acid load is a great way to predict stone formation. Basically, when you add more nutrient rich and alkalizing foods, you could reduce the stone promoters from getting bigger.

Eating a diet heavy in acidic foods can increase metabolic acidosis and this in turn can increase the risk of kidney disease. One study followed over 15,000 people who didn't have kidney disease for 21 years. These people were already at a high risk for developing atherosclerosis. After they adjusted for factors such as demographics and caloric intake, they found that participants who consumed foods that were more acidic had a higher risk of developing chronic kidney disease.

Some of the dietary components like getting protein from vegetable sources and a higher intake of magnesium protected against chronic kidney disease.

- Chronic low back pain

Research is still being done on this but there is a bit of evidence that indicates that chronic back pain could improve by adding in a supplement of alkalizing minerals. Increasing magnesium by taking supplements helps the enzyme system function better and activates vitamin D. This will, in turn, improve your back pain. Basically, if you have back pain, following the alkaline diet will give your level of magnesium a boost and might ease your symptoms.

- Type 2 diabetes

Around tenth of the adult population within the U.S. has been diagnosed with a kind of a pair of polygenic disease (Type 2 diabetes). This is an upset that may cause your glucose to rise. This can cause your cells to become resistant to insulin. Type two polygenic disorder is preventable and analysis has shown that dietary acid load has been related to multiplied risk. Basically, it has also been shown that in addition to helping you keep a healthy weight, a diet that promotes alkaline foods might cut back the danger of developing type 2 of the polygenic disorder.

During a study in Germany in 2014, researchers followed 66,485 women for 14 years prior. Within that time there was 1,372 new cases of diabetes that was diagnosed. The researchers analyzed their food intake and determined that the women who ate diet that were high in acid based foods had higher risks of developing diabetes. The researchers suggest that high intake of foods that are acidic might be linked to insulin resistance which has been linked to diabetes.

- Osteoporosis

Osteoporosis is a progressive bone disease that is characterized by a lower than normal bone mineral content. This is a common problem for postmenopausal women and will dramatically increase a person's risk of fractures. It is believed that in order to keep your blood pH constant, the body will start to take alkaline minerals, like calcium, out of the bones to buffer the excess acids when excessive acid-forming foods are consumed.

According to this believe, acid-forming diets, like that standard Western diet, will end up causing a los in bone density. This is what they refer to as "acid-ash hypothesis of osteoporosis." However, there is one problem with this theory, it leaves out the function of the kidneys, which play an important part in removing acids from the body and regulates body pH. The kidneys make what is known as bicarbonate ions that help to neutralize acids that are in your blood to help the body closely mange the pH of the blood.

The respiratory system also kicks into action when there are excess acid levels. When the bicarbonate ions that your kidneys produce binds to the acids within your blood, they create what is known as carbon dioxide, which is then breathed that out, and water, which is excreted. This theory also ignores that the main cause of osteoporosis is a loss in the protein collagen within the bones. Ironically, having a loss in collagen has often been linked to low levels of ascorbic acid and orthosilicic acid.

It's important that you keep in mind that scientific evident that links dietary acid to bone density or fracture risk is a mixed bag. While there have been many observational studies that haven't found any association, others have found many significant links. Clinical trials, which are often the most accurate, have found that acid-forming diets don't have a large impact on calcium levels within the body.

While scientific studies may be mixed, there are still plenty of people who say the standard Western diet does impose a high acid load, which can affect bone health. To lower this risk of osteoporosis, it is important that people consume seven to nine servings of vegetables and fruits each day to help keep the pH balanced so that the body never feels it necessary to take calcium from the bones.

- Muscle mass

When we age, we will lose muscle mass, and it will be more prominent if you lead an inactive lifestyle. Having less muscle mass will mean you burn fewer calories throughout the day and this contributes to that "weight creep" that many people will develop as they age. Losing muscle mass will make you more susceptible to fracturing a bone if we fall and this could hinder your independence. A diet rich in alkaline vegetables and fruits can reduce the net acid load in older adults this can result in preserving muscle mass. Basically, everybody wants their independence when aging and adding in a serving of vegetables and fruits to every meal could help.

During a three year research that involved 384 women and men that were aged 65 and older showed that eating a lot of foods that are rich in potassium like fresh vegetables and fruits might help adults maintain their muscle mass as they age. In recent studies, researchers looked at data collected in 2013 from a group of 2,689 women who were aged from 18 to 79 and found a significant association between following the alkaline diet and keeping muscle mass. A diet rich in alkaline vegetables and fruits can reduce the net acid load in older adults this can result in preserving muscle mass. Basically, everybody wants their independence when aging and adding in a serving of vegetables and fruits to every meal could help.

- Chemotherapy and cancer

Even though acidosis caused by diet could increase the risk for cancer, right now there isn't any research that the alkaline could prevent cancer. Some studies have shown that when you eat more foods that promote alkalinity, the pH in the urine could be changed to help how effective chemotherapy drugs work. If you been diagnosed with cancer and are taking chemotherapy, talk with your doctor or dietitian before changing your diet. Basically, it would be best if you eat a diet that has an emphasis on plant foods, consuming between five and nine servings of vegetables and fruits every day, and don't consume a lot of red meat, processed meats, alcohol, and sodium which is a lot like the alkaline diet.

A normal American diet leaves a lot to be desired and this leaves our bodies short of many essential minerals and vitamins. If this is left unchecked, for a short amount of time, it could make you feel tired, cause weight gain, change your concentration levels and mood, and disrupt sleep. For longer amounts of your time, imbalances within the diet may cause chronic diseases like kidney stones, heart condition, type two polygenic disease, and high-pressure level. Giving your body a mixture of nutrient-dense foods daily will give it a chance to fight against the disease.

If you have been diagnosed with any health conditions like cancer or kidney disease, make sure you talk with your health care provider before changing your diet. If you take medicines that change how the body absorbs potassium, calcium, or other minerals you need to check with your doctor before starting this diet.

Following the food list too strictly without taking into consideration factors such as overall calorie intake or protein could cause other health problems such as excessive weight loss or nutrient deficiency.

An alkaline diet should never be used instead of normal treatment for any health problem, adopting a diet that is rich in vegetables and fruits might help protect you against specific diseases and have better health overall.

There are many foods on the foods list such as nuts, beans, and grains that have great attributes and then the foods such as wine and coffee need to be consumed in moderation. Instead of looking at the foods as ones to eat and what to avoid, think about the base and acid forming foods and try to have a balanced diet.

80/20 Rule

When you decide to get healthy, you can't expect to be perfect on the first day and you can't deprive yourself of foods that you really enjoy. To have success when learning to eat alkaline and keeping this lifestyle, you need to learn moderation since life is about balance. Deprivation is the reason behind the failures of most diets. Finding the perfect balance can be confusing and challenging when you first begin this new lifestyle. In order to get the most benefits out of the alkaline diet is to use the 80/20 rule. This means that in order to keep a healthy internal environment, you need to try to eat a diet that contains around 80 percent alkaline-forming foods and the remaining 20 percent coming from acid-forming foods. Basically, refined starches and animal proteins are acid, whereas, fruits, vegetables, and beans are alkaline.

It is easy to put this into play if you just visualize your plate and think about food groups. To have optimal health, you need to eat plant proteins, healthy fats, tubers, vegetables, and fruits that take up 80 percent of your plate. Other acidic foods and starches will take the remaining 20 percent. If you can do this for every meal, this will guarantee your diet will always be 80 percent alkaline and 20 percent acid. You might be tempted to get rid of all alkaline foods from your diet. This would be a huge mistake. High protein foods like beans, fish, milk, and meat are acidifying but your body has to have protein so it can repair and rebuild your body.

If you like tofu that is mildly alkaline and low acid then go ahead and put it into your diet. Just eat it in moderation. Even though it isn't a high protein food, you can even have a piece of chocolate or a slice of birthday cake every now and then. The key words are moderation, balance, and shifting your diet from constantly eating acid-forming foods to a diet where they begin taking up a small part of your plate. Slowly bring back in foods that have the most impact and before you realize what is happening, all that good will outweigh the bad and your energy and health will increase.

Exercise

Another essential component to help manage stress, keeping a healthy weight, and decreasing the risk of chronic disease is physical activity. Here is a guideline for persons over six years old:

- Adolescents and Children

  - Adolescents and children need to include bone and muscle-strengthening activities for one hour each day for three days per week.

  - One hour a day needs to be either vigorous or moderate-intensity aerobic activity. There should be a vigorous activity done three days per week.

  - Adolescents and children need to perform one hour or more of physical activity each day.

- Adults

  - For substantial advantages, adults have to do about seventy-five minutes per week of vigorous intensity or no less than a hundred and fifty minutes per week of moderate-intensity exercise or an equal combination of these two. Aerobic exercises need to be performed in a series of ten minutes intervals.

- For in-depth benefits, adults have to increase their aerobic activity to three hundred minutes per week or one hundred fifty minutes of vigorous intensity activity per week.

- Adults have to do muscle-strengthening activities that involve each major muscle cluster for 2 days or a lot weekly.

- Older Adults

  - If an older adult can't do a hundred and fifty minutes per week of moderate-intensity activity because of chronic conditions, they need to be physically active if their conditions and ability allow it.

While we all know that we need to exercise, we may not completely understand why we should and what it can do for us. Let's take a look at some of the many benefits regular exercise can provide:

1. It can increase your energy levels – Exercise is able to improve both the efficiency and strength of your cardiovascular system to help send nutrients and oxygen to your muscles. When the cardiovascular systems works more efficiently, everything else seems easier and you will find that you have more energy for the things you enjoy doing.

2. It can improve your muscle strength – When you stay active, it keeps your muscles strong and your ligaments, joints, and tendons flexible. This allows you to move more easily and keeps you from injuring yourself. When you have strong ligaments and muscles, you help to reduce your risk of lower back and joint pain by keeping everything in proper alignment. This will also end up improving your balance and coordination.

3. It helps you to keep a healthy weight – Exercise helps you to burn calories. In addition, the more muscle mass you have, you will increase your metabolic rate. This means that you burn more calories at rest. This will help to boost your self-esteem and help you to lose weight.

4. It improves the function of the brain – Exercise improves your oxygen levels and blood flow to the brain. It will also encourage the release of hormones that help with the production of cells within the hippocampus, which is the area of the brain that helps with learning and memory. This will then help to boost your cognitive ability and concentration level, and it lowers you risk of cognitive degenerative diseases like Alzheimer's

5. It helps your heart – Exercise helps to your reduce your LDL levels, which is what clogs your arteries. It increases your HDL levels and lowers your blood pressure, so the stress on your heart is reduced. It also helps to strengthen the muscles of your heart. When you combine this with a healthy diet, exercise is able to lower your risk of coronary heart disease.

6. It lowers your risk for type 2 diabetes – Exercising regularly helps keep your blood glucose levels under control, which delays or prevents the onset of diabetes. Exercise will also help to prevent obesity, which is the main factor in diabetes.

7. Improves the immune system – Exercise helps the body to pump oxygen and nutrients through the body that it needs to help fuel the cells that fight off viruses and bacteria.

8. It helps to reduce the chance of developing degenerative bone disease – Exercises that are weight bearing, like weight training, walking, or running, helps to lower your risk of osteoporosis and osteoarthritis.

9. It can help to reduce some cancers – Being fit could mean that it could reduce your risk of breast cancer, colon cancer, and maybe even lung and endometrial cancers. According to studies performed by Seattle Cancer Research Center, they suggest that 35% of all cancer related deaths were linked to being sedentary and overweight.

10. It helps you sleep better – Being physically active makes you tired, thus, you will be ready for bed. Having good sleep quality helps to improve your overall wellness and it can help to reduce stress.

11. You will have a better mood and wellbeing – Exercise is able to help stimulate the release of endorphins which will make you feel even better and feel relaxed. These endorphins will also work to improve your mood and lower stress.

12. It can help treat or prevent mental illness – Exercise has the power to help your meet others, lower stress, provides you a sense of achievement, cope with frustration, and provide you with that all important "me time," all of this can help you prevent depression.

Advantages

Here is a rundown of all the advantages the alkaline diet offers your body:

- It can increase your sex drive and enhances sexual power.

- It can slow down the natural aging process and will keep you looking fresher and younger.

- It can improve the health of your teeth and gums.

- The alkaline diet can increase your body's available energy and will keep it energized throughout the day.

- It will help you lose weight.

- It can help improve your body's immunity and can protect you from developing cancer.

- It can help boost how the body absorbs vitamins and minimizes the deficiency of magnesium.

- It can help lower chronic pain and inflammation.

- It will lower the risk of stroke and hypertension.

- It can help protect bone mass and muscle density.

Foods and Your Body

Scientists have known for some time now that what makes up our diets can affect the acid balance in our bodies. Changes in the acidity of your urine that are brought on by changes in your diet have always been interesting to physiologists. This shows the role kidneys play in maintaining homeostasis or the state of balance within our bodies. Research from the Paleolithic era shows the drastic changes in the diet as compared to ones of our ancestors who were hunter-gatherers and the rise of chronic diseases.

Michael Pollan's guideline of "Eat food, not too much, mostly plants" is quoted often but isn't followed that often. Most of

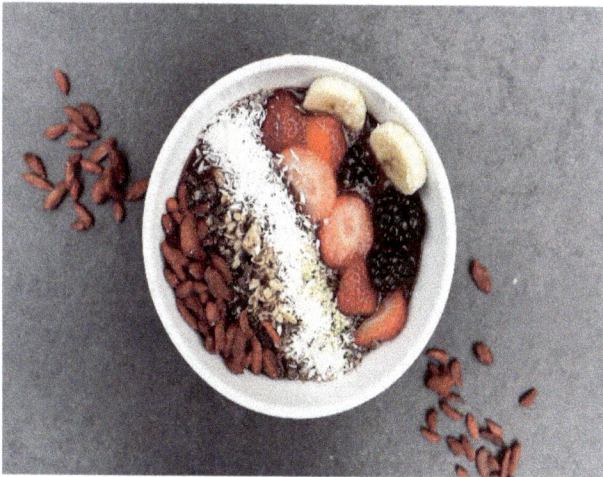

the Americans' calories come from processed foods that don't have any valuable nutrients but are extremely high in unhealthy fats, added sugars, and sodium. These foods are coupled with large amounts of animal proteins and very low intake of vegetables and fruits. It isn't a surprise that this diet causes diseases but we don't know why. One reason is the modern diet exchanged magnesium and potassium-rich foods for salt. This creates a deficiency of potassium within the diet and this increases the acid load inside the body.

What's worse is with time, a diet high in acid will produce a "low grade chronic metabolic acidosis". This means we are constantly in a state of inflammation and high acidity. Since our bodies have to operate in a stable pH, it has to neutralize a very high dietary acid load that puts a strain on our body's buffering system. The consequences for our body constantly attempting to keep a constant pH within the high acidic environment will lead to wasting muscle and increased chronic diseases.

Acute inflammation like our bodies responding to a cut or fever is necessary for health. Chronic inflammation, on the other hand, is a normal process that has gone very wrong. It has a domino effect that could seriously undermine our health. Good news is, what you put in your mouth will affect your inflammation levels. Eating foods like spices and herbs will help reduce the inflammation in the body and this is the best way to protect your health.

When you can lower the acid-producing foods in your diet and replace it with alkaline-producing foods, this can lower acid levels and will reduce the strain on our body's natural buffering system. Reducing the acid load in the body might delay or prevent kidney stones from forming, improve heart health by promoting a healthier blood pressure, lowering your risk for type 2 diabetes, and maintaining muscle mass. Employing some strategies to help neutralize your diet might mean a difference between a healthy, disease-free body and chronic low-grade acidosis.

Alkaline Water

You might have heard about alkaline water. This type of water is less acidic than even tap water and it is a lot better. Alkaline water is rich in bicarbonate, magnesium, potassium, silica, and calcium. Normal tap water is normally neutral. It has a pH of about seven. Alkaline water will have a pH of about eight or nine. Alkaline water can be found at most grocery stores, and you can find water ionizer in many large chain stores, too. Regular water is great for the majority of people since there isn't scientific evidence that verifies all the claims that alkaline water brags about. The current research claiming alkaline water can help treat chronic acidosis, reduces liver damage, improves gut health, protects from toxins, improves health overall, is not convincing. It is also believed to help slow down the ageing process and keep your pH levels regulated.

To get alkaline water, regular water has to go through ionization process. This process increases the pH level of the water. There are many different ways you can increase the alkaline properties in your water by using additives, faucet attachments, and filters. These are things you can do at home which may be cheaper than buying bottled alkaline water. In a study published in the *Annals of Otology, Rhinology & Laryngology*, alkaline water that has a pH of 8.8 could actually help soothe acid reflux symptoms because the acid is due to high levels of pepsin, and the pH of alkaline water has the ability to kill the enzyme. Pepsin, by the way, is a natural enzyme that the body uses to break down food proteins. In another study published in the *Journal of the International Society of Sports Nutrition* has found a significant different in the blood viscosity in those who consumed high pH water as compared to regular water after a strenuous workout. In yet another study, this one published in the *Shanghai Journal of Preventive Medicine,* found that alkaline water could benefit those who suffer from diabetes, high cholesterol, and high blood pressure.

It's possible that drinking alkaline water could provide some benefits for some, but studies haven't produced evidence that it will benefit your health. People who have kidney disease or who take specific medications that change the function of the kidneys are cautioned against it since the minerals in alkaline water might add up in the body. If you don't have kidney problems, you might think about drinking alkaline water. Water that has naturally occurring minerals will be your best bet as a source for alkaline water.

While there may not be a large amount of proven scientific research concerning alkaline water, there is still many proponents who believe that alkaline water can provide you with the following:

1. Alkaline water has better hydrating properties than normal tap water. This makes it beneficial for people who work out regularly and need more water in their body. From a scientific viewpoint, the water molecules within alkaline

water are smaller and your cells are able to more easily absorb them, which helps to re-hydrate the body.

2. Alkaline water can also boost your immunity. Having a healthy immune system can help to neutralize the acidity in your body, which can be caused by environmental toxins, stress, and a poor diet.

3. Alkaline water also contains different minerals like calcium and magnesium, both of which are extremely important for keeping your bones healthy.

4. Alkaline water also contains potent antioxidants that help to stop the growth of cell damaging free radicals within the body, which can increase the ageing process.

5. One of the best benefits of drinking alkaline water is that it can help to neutralize the acidity in the body by lowering the excessive acid content in the gastrointestinal tract and the stomach.

If you want to start consuming alkaline water, you don't have to go to the store and buy packages of the expensive alkaline water. You can make your own right at home. You can use baking soda to make you own alkaline water. Baking soda has a pH of 9. Mix in a half of a tablespoon of baking soda to a gallon of water. Shake it to make sure that the baking soda dissolves. Once dissolves, enjoy a cup. Make sure you stick to these measurements. While baking soda is good for you, you can overdose on it.

You can also make alkaline water using lemon. While lemon is considered acidic with a pH below 7, when it is added to water, or consumed and metabolized, it has an alkalizing effect and raises the body's pH. This is why you should always kick start you day with a glass of lemon water. There is no right or wrong way with this one. Add as much lemon juice as you like to your water and enjoy.

Alkaline Foods

There are many foods that are easy to tell whether they belong in the alkaline or acid category but there are also foods that are so evident. Let's look at a lemon. A lemon has a very tart taste so it is obviously acidic. Wrong, the nature of lemon is acidic, when the body metabolizes it, it becomes alkalizing. Foods that have a natural acidity don't always remain acidic once they have been eaten. Acidic foods such as sauerkraut, kefir, and citrus are alkalizing and very healing. What makes it even more confusing, many charts that show alkalizing and acidifying foods just use the words "alkaline foods" and "acid foods". This doesn't give an accurate picture in any way. In order to be able to accurately predict the base or acid potential of any food, scientists have worked a long time to come up with a technique that uses the food's nutrient composition and determines what the baseload or true acid that goes into our bodies.

This brought about the PRAL or potential renal acid load scale. A PRAL score that is negative shows food that is alkaline or basic. If the PRAL score is positive, it shows that the foods are acidic. If the score shows zero, the food will be neutral. If the score is negative, then the food is alkaline. If you add up the PRAL values for every food that you eat during the day, you will get your net alkaline or acid load. While it isn't necessary to micromanage your diet to find the lowest PRAL score, it might be interesting to figure out your PRAL values are on any given day.

To example this further, PRAL measures the acidity or alkalinity of a food based on the amount of phosphorus, minerals, and protein that is leaves behind within the body once your body has metabolized it. Since phosphorus and protein break down into phosphoric acid and sulfuric acid, they believe to be acidifying to the body. When you metabolize an alkaline food, it leaves behind trace amounts of alkaline minerals, like potassium, magnesium, and calcium.

Here is a list of foods and their PRAL score to give you an idea of what this all means:

- Fruits:

    o Watermelon : -1.9

    o Strawberries: -2.2

    o Raisins: -21

    o Pineapple: -2.7

- Pear: -2.9

- Peach: -2.4

- Orange: -2.7

- Mango: -3.3

- Lemon: -2.6

- Kiwi fruit: -4.1

- Grapes: -3.9

- Grapefruit: -3.5

- Dried figs: -18.1

- Cherries: -3.6

- Black currants: -6.5

- Bananas: -5.5

- Apricots: -4.8

- Apples: -2.2

- Fish & Seafood

  - Zander: 7.1

  - Trout: 10.8

  - Tiger prawn: 18.2

  - Sole: 7.4

- o Shrimp: 7.6

- o Sardines: 13.5

- o Herring: 8

- o Salmon: 9.4

- o Rose-fish: 10

- o Prawn: 15.3

- o Mussels: 15.3

- o Halibut: 7.8

- o Eel: 11

- o Cod: 7.1

- o Carp: 7.9

- **Nuts**

  - o Walnuts: 6.8

  - o Sweet almonds: 4.3

  - o Pistachio: 8.5

  - o Peanuts: 8.3

  - o Hazelnuts: -2.8

- **Fats & Oil**

  - o Sunflower seed oil: 0

- o   Olive oil: 0

- o   Margarine: -0.5

- o   Butter: 0.6

- **Beverages**

  - o   Dry white wine: -1.2

  - o   Vegetable juice: -3.6

  - o   Tomato juice: -2.8

  - o   Tea: -0.3

  - o   Red wine: -2.4

  - o   Unsweetened orange juice: -2.9

  - o   Mineral water: -0.1

  - o   Lemon juice: -2.5

  - o   Herbal tea: -0.2

  - o   Green tea: -0.3

  - o   Unsweetened grape juice: -1

  - o   Fruit tea: -0.3

  - o   Espresso: -2.3

  - o   Coffee: -1.4

  - o   Cocoa with semi-skimmed milk: -0.4

- Coca-cola: 0.4

- Carrot juice: -4.8

- Beetroot juice: -3.9

- Beer, stout: -0.1

- Beer, pale: 0.9

- Beer, draft: -0.2

- Unsweetened apple juice: -2.2

- Grains

  - Wheat flour: 6.9

  - Rye flour: 5.9

  - Rice, white: 1.7

  - Rice, brown: 12.5

  - Millet: 8.6

  - Corn: 3.9

- Bread

  - White bread: 3.7

  - Pumpernickel: 4.2

- Dairy Products and Eggs

  - Whey: -1.6

- Kefir: 0

- Parmesan: 34.2

- Plain yogurt: 1.5

- Gouda: 18.6

- Egg: 8.2

- Meats

  - Lean beef: 7.8

  - Chicken: 8.7

  - Duck: 4.1

  - Goose: 13

  - Pork sausage: 7

  - Salami: 11.6

  - Turkey: 9.9

- Sweets

  - White sugar: 0

  - Brown sugar: -1.2

  - Milk chocolate: 2.4

  - Honey: -0.3

- Veggies

- o Onions: -1.5

- o Brussels sprouts: -4.5

- o Garlic: -1.7

- o Potatoes: -4

- o Soy beans: -3.4

- o Mushrooms: -1.4

- o Lettuce: -2.5

- o Kohlrabi: -5.5

- o Zucchini: -4.6

- Herbs & Vinegar

  - o Parsley: -12

  - o Apple cider vinegar: -2.3

  - o Basil: -7.3

  - o Chives: -5.3

As you can see, the foods that rank most alkaline on this scale are the veggies and fruits, and one nut. The foods that are most acidic are poultry, eggs, grains, seafood, and dairy products.

I really hate to be the bearer of bad news, but parmesan cheese ranks at +34.2 on the PRAL scale. This means that it is one of the most acidifying foods in the standard diet. Now, you may be wondering how on Earth dairy could be acidic since it contains calcium, which is one of the alkaline minerals. The reason for the acidity in dairy is due to its phosphorus content. It contains more phosphorus than it does calcium, making it acidic.

A quick note to make sure there isn't any confusing, the PRAL table measures the acidity of food in a different way to than how the pH of your blood is measured.

If we were to look at the PRAL scores on a regular pH scale, the 7.8 score of beef would mean that it is alkaline or neutral instead of acidic. Unlike the pH scale that we talked about earlier, a food on the PRAL scale that has a negative score actually means that it has more alkaline producing properties.

Foods to Avoid

When you want to restore the balance of pH in your body, you have to know what foods to eat and the ones to stay away from. A food's tendency to form acid in our bodies doesn't have anything to do with the food's natural pH. Instead, foods get classified according to the minerals that they release into the urine. When you are beginning, use the list below to help you decide about which of these foods you want to include into your 20 percent or stay away from them totally.

- Sodium

It is recommended that Americans only consume 2,300 milligrams of sodium or less each day. Just about anyone could benefit from less sodium in their diet because of its negative impact on our hearts. Sodium can be sneaky. It shows up in the majority of the foods we consume each day even if you don't shake a saltshaker. Since it is acid-forming, try to find unprocessed fresh foods that will keep your sodium low.

- Alcohol

Just a small amount of alcohol will have an effect on your body. Once you drink, the alcohol gets absorbed into the bloodstream and goes all through the body where it stays until the liver has time to process it. Out of the four macronutrients, only three of them can be stored in the body. These are fat, carbohydrates, and protein. The fourth one, alcohol, can't. For this reason alone, it will take priority over everything to be metabolized. When the body does this, all the other processes that need to take place get interrupted. Alcohol doesn't have any nutrients and is looked at as toxic waste by the body and should only be consumed in moderation.

- Grains

The grains that are consumed the most in the United States are wheat and corn. Both of these are very acidic. Once they are consumed and the body metabolizes them, they will produce acids that the liver has to get rid of. Wheat contains gluten which is a protein that many people with celiac disease or gluten intolerance can't digest. Since this protein can't get broken down, the body will attack it like an allergen and this can cause cramping, bloating, and gas. All grains are not equal. Some are alkaline like wild rice, quinoa, millet, and amaranth. Most of the grains that Americans eat are in products made with corn or refined flour. Refined grains don't have any fiber or vitamin B and are very high-glycemic foods. These could cause spikes in your blood sugar and makes your body store fat.

- Caffeine

Have you ever stopped to think about what goes into your body when you sip coffee or drink that energy drink? Caffeine, just like alcohol, gets into the bloodstream fast and it will take 45 minutes for about 99 percent of the caffeine to get absorbed through the membranes of the stomach, throat, and mouth. Caffeine is considered basic but cola, hot chocolate, energy drinks, tea, and coffee are acid-forming because there are other chemicals in play like acetic acid, formic acid, and phosphorus. Once it has been absorbed, the liver will metabolize caffeine and the by-products get filtered by the kidneys and leave the body through urine. To lessen the stress on your liver, try to switch your normal coffee for herbal tea or a glass of water.

- Refined sugar

Americans consume way too much sugar, and just like sodium, it is found in most of the foods we eat. A normal American will consume around 22 teaspoons of sugar daily. This can add up to more than 70 pounds each year. The current recommendation for adding sugar is no more than five teaspoons daily for women and between eight and nine teaspoons daily for men. Consuming too much sugar could lead to high cholesterol, diabetes, high blood sugar, and unhealthy weight gain. The biggest sources of added sugars are foods like dairy, desserts, cookies, cakes, candy, and soft drinks. Look at the nutrition label on foods to find out how much sugar is in the foods you consume daily. Fresh whole foods don't contain added sugar; try to stick with eating natural foods that contain nutrient-rich sugars the way nature intended it to be.

- Animal products

The highest acid-forming foods you eat are found in dairy, eggs, and meat. In the United States, people eat way too much animal products. They make it the center point of the meal instead of using it as a side. Animal proteins, if they aren't organic, could contain antibiotics and hormones. Animal proteins are high in cholesterol and saturated fats. Eggs and meat contain many sulfur-containing amino acids that get metabolized into sulfuric acid and has to be buffered by the body by using calcium compounds and this puts more strain on the kidneys. Your body has to have sufficient protein to recover and repair the body, so you can't get rid of protein entirely. You need to balance out your choices and use ones that are alkaline-forming. With the alkaline diet, you are going to get a lot of nutrient-rich, fiber-packed plant proteins by swapping meat for legumes and beans a couple times each week.

Foods to Enjoy

Good news is that there isn't a shortage of alkalizing foods that feed our bodies with lots of antioxidants, phytochemicals, minerals, and vitamins that will improve your health and add vitality. Use the following foods to find all the health benefits for the foods that are allowed on this diet. Focus on the foods you can add instead of what you should get rid of or reduce. Making a subtle shift in the way you think can make a huge difference. It can remove judgment, anxiety, and stress. Eat the good foods first and you might realize there isn't any room left for bad stuff.

- Nightshades – PRAL -8.6

Members of the common nightshade family include hot chili peppers, sweet bell peppers, tomatoes, eggplant, white potatoes, and any spice that is made from peppers like cayenne pepper, red pepper flakes, and paprika. This is a small list but it contains a large number of important benefits. Tomatoes are a good source of lycopene which is a phytochemical. This can lower your risk of developing prostate cancer. Capsaicin, which is a compound found in peppers, is a powerful anti-inflammatory for the body. All these foods are high in fiber, vitamin C, and other minerals including magnesium and potassium.

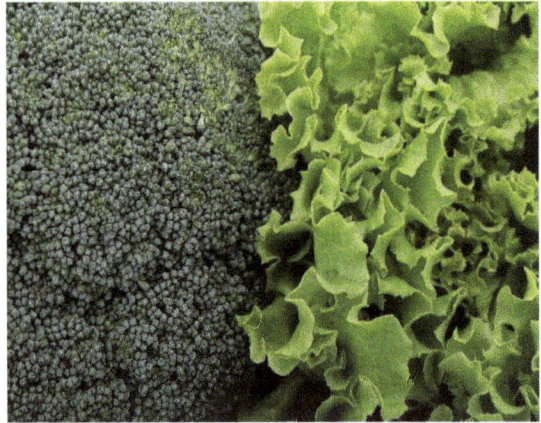

- Eggplant – PRAL -3.4

Besides the fact that it is alkaline, eggplants is a food that offers phytonutrients like chlorogenic acid. This acid is not acidifying to the body, instead, it is a plant compound that helps aid your metabolism and digestion. Eggplants are also delicious when you bake it in some olive oil, added to salads, or used as a pizza crust.

- Pears – PRAL -2.9

Pears have high fiber content and low sugar content, which is a great fruit even for people who suffer from blood sugar imbalances. Pears also have a lot of vitamin C content, which is great for protecting your cells from carcinogens.

- Beet Greens – PRAL -16.7

Let's hear it for the most alkaline food in the world: beet greens. While beet greens may not be one of the most popular greens in our currently diet, their amazing alkalinity score makes them a great choice to add into stir-fries or smoothies. Besides the fact that they have a high alkaline content, beet greens are also slightly bitter that could end up helping stimulate bile productions in order to help you digest fats better.

If this doesn't give you enough of a reason to stops throwing out your beet tops, I don't know what will. Beet greens can be used to replace any type of greens you use in smoothies, soups, or salads.

- Hazelnuts – PRAL -2.8

The majority of nuts come with an acidifying effect, but hazelnuts have proven to be the exception to the rule. So if you enjoy nuts, these are the best choice to include into your daily diet in comparison to peanuts, which have a score of +8 and are highly acidic to your body. Hazelnuts are famous for their contribution to nut butters, such as Nutella, but your make your own version of this that is healthy if you enjoy this particular spread.

- Pineapple – PRAL -2.7

Pineapple is very alkalizing and delicious, plus they are good for your digestion, so much so, several dietary supplements add them to digestive-boosting formulas. This is due to the fact that pineapples contain a digestive enzyme known as bromelain. Bromelain is also believed to be helpful in killing of intestinal parasites.

- Leafy greens – PRAL -11.8

Leafy green vegetables are the most nutritious foods that you could eat. It doesn't matter if you put them into a smoothie or eat them as a salad; these are very alkalizing and high in phytochemicals and nutrients. Yes, all greens are nutritious, but some of the top choices for maximum health include mustard greens, arugula, turnip greens, Swiss chard, spinach, and kale. Greens are nutritional powerhouses and are high in fiber. They don't have many calories and contain lots of vitamin K and calcium for bone health. Greens are also high in vitamins C and A, potassium, along with zeaxanthin and lutein. Studies show that the phytochemicals and carotenoids in folate greens might help reduce the risk of certain cancers, helps with managing weight, and lowers the chance of type 2 polygenic disease.

Spinach, specifically, is also for its bone health properties because of its calcium content. Because it is highly alkalizing, anti-cancer juicing protocols will often include spinach into their regimen.

- Kale – PRAL -8.3

People don't refer kale as the new beef for nothing. Kale is high in vitamin K, calcium, and iron, which is believed to be a great protector against many forms of cancer. Besides all of these benefits, kale is another extremely alkaline food. Kale is mild in taste and you can add it into any recipes to help jazz it up. Kale can easily be added into recipes that call for greens, or in soups, salads and stir fires.

- Swiss Chard – PRAL -8.1

Have you started to see a trend here? Some of the world's most alkaline foods are leafy greens. Swiss chard is just another green that can provide you with a whole lot of nutritious benefits with vitamins that help to support our cellular health, like vitamin K. Swiss chard also has plant protein and phosphorus, but the PRAL score tells us that it leaves behind more alkalizing minerals than it does acidity when the body metabolizes it. Swiss chard is great to use as the wrap for a lettuce wrap in any recipe that calls for a tortilla or any sort of grain bread.

- Squashes – PRAL -8.6 to -6.0

Squash is an umbrella term that covers many types of vegetables that include winter squashes like cushaw, butternut, Hubbard, and acorn, summer varieties like crookneck and zucchini, and pumpkins. Squash is very versatile and can be substituted for noodles, julienned, or put into stir-fries or salads. Squashes are high in vitamin A, E, B, and C along with the minerals iron, calcium, potassium, and magnesium. Adding squash into your diet could keep your heart healthy due to the potassium. It also lowers inflammation by providing the phytochemicals beta-carotene, zeaxanthin, and lutein. It protects against certain cancers by adding carotenoids and vitamin A.

- Bananas – PRAL -6.9

Bananas, or as I like to call them, potassium sticks, are another great food to eat that is highly alkalizing, plus, it's also delicious. Bananas are a perfect source of fiber, which will help to promote your digestive regularity and get rid of any toxins within your gastrointestinal tract. You eat enough bananas; your colon won't be missing those grains. While a lot of people want to stay away from bananas when they are trying to lose weight because of their sugar content, eating a banana is a lot better for you than grabbing a handful of granola or some other pre-packaged processed food that is full of unhealthy sugars and acidifying ingredients.

One of the best ways you can add more bananas to your diet is to use it to make ice cream. All you have to do is freeze peeled bananas and then blend them up until they form a creamy consistency. The part is that you can add in other alkalizing foods to change up the flavor, like berries and mint.

- Zucchini – PRAL -2.6

Zucchini contains lutein, which is a great source of phytonutrients. Lutein is part of the same category of antioxidants as beta-carotene, which means that it can help with eye health. Zucchini has carved itself a niche in the diet world as being a vegan, gluten-free, low-carb pasta alternative. A spiralizer can be used to make zucchini pasta noodles, know lovingly as zoodles. Toss them in your favorite alkaline pasta sauce, and you have a delicious meal.

- Strawberries – PRAL -2.2

Strawberries are another great source of vitamin C. They also have a high manganese contain, which is a trace mineral that the body needs to help facilitate metabolic function. There are an endless number of ways to enjoy strawberries.

- Apples – PRAL -2.2

Apples have long been viewed as one of the healthiest foods in the world, mainly because they have a high content of detoxifying fiber and vitamin C, as well as flavonoids that help to fight off cancer. These are all essential nutrients for the body and help to promote healthy cholesterol and blood pressure levels. To get even more health benefits from these delicious foods, it's a good idea to add apple cider vinegar to your daily diet. When apples are fermented to make vinegar, they contain a nutrient known as acetic acid, which provides antiviral and antibacterial benefits. If you're not a fan of the taste of apple cider vinegar, whether diluted or not, that's fine, there are many other ways you can use apple cider vinegar without having to taste it.

- Lentils and beans – PRAL -14.4 to 8.6

Legumes and beans are full of nutritious things. Packed in each bean is potassium, iron, B vitamins, fiber, little to no sodium or fat, and plant proteins that are heart healthy. Beans can lower the risk for cancer and heart disease because all the many different phytochemicals that are present. Beans lower cholesterol because they give the body soluble fiber. This is the same fiber that helps you feel full and keeps your glucose steady. Some choices in this group are acidic but they aren't as acidifying as animal proteins. The best beans to choose are yellow and green like split peas, lima beans, pigeon peas, black beans, and kidney beans.

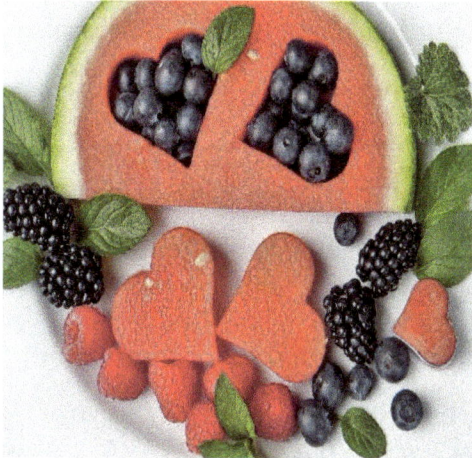

- Watermelon – PRAL -1.9

Watermelon is another healthy alkalizing food that can help to provide you body with important electrolytes to aid in cardiac function, like potassium. Since watermelons are made up of mostly water, they also keep you hydrated more so than any other vegetables and fruits. Watermelon is a delicious snack, but you can also have fun and get creative with it.

- Crucifers – PRAL -1.2 to -4.9

This is the most nutritious group of foods. When talking about nutrients, their states are extremely high in vitamins C and A, fiber, folic acid, and carotenoids. Collards and kale are technically leafy greens but are cruciferous vegetables and contain more vitamin K than all other vegetables. The phytochemical content of these vegetables can lower the risk of developing certain cancers including breast, lung, colorectal, and prostate. They are low in calories and are alkaline-forming. In order to get all their benefits, try to consume one to two cups each day. There is a lot to choose from such as cauliflower, bok choy, kale, collard greens, cabbage, Brussels sprouts, and broccoli.

Cauliflower is an amazing alkaline food that can help to aid in rebalancing your hormones when the estrogen levels in your body are too high. This is due to the fact that cauliflower contains what is call Indole-3-Carbinol, which helps your body to regular estrogen levels. We all come in contact with estrogen regularly through foods that contain estrogen, like soy, chemicals within our environment, like plastics, and pharmaceutical drugs, like oral contraceptives. Too much estrogen within then body is very harmful to the body and can cause digestive problems like bloating, weight gain, and can cause infertility and reproductive cancers.

- Cherries – PRAL -3.6

Cherries have already made a name for themselves as one of the best sources of antioxidants like anthocyanins, which help to reduce your cancer risk. Studies have also found that cherries are great at relieving inflammation linked to arthritis and joint pain, and could even help to prevent cardiovascular disease. Cherries can easily be added to smoothies. When you have a post-workout shake, you want to make sure it includes plenty of alkaline foods. This is due to the fact that lactic acid, which is a substance that naturally helps to improve your body's energy, is released naturally during an intense exercise. As you can guess by its name, lactic acid will make the body more acidic, which is the reason for consuming alkaline foods after a workout to help neutralize the acids.

- Seeds and nuts – PRAL -1.4

For some people, some of their favorite nuts could be moderately acid-forming like pecans, peanuts, hazelnuts, and walnuts. There are still a lot of varieties of seeds and nuts you can eat that will have alkalizing effects on the body. Chestnuts are among the most alkaline-forming nut because of their water content. The next is almonds that are second on the alkaline scale. Nuts, even the ones that are slightly acidic still contain vitamin E, zinc, magnesium, fiber, and healthy fats. Seeds that you can eat while following the alkaline diet include sunflower, sesame, flax, hemp, and chia. Adding nuts as a part of your healthy diet can bring benefits to your heart, add nutrients, and help weight management by making you feel fuller longer.

- Celery – PRAL -5.2

Aside from the fact that it is alkalizing, celery also comes along with some cleansing properties. Since it is made up of mostly water, celery is able to flush toxins from the body. Celery is also one of those magic "negative calorie" foods. This means that when you eat celery, it will require your body to burn more calories to chew and digest it than it actually contains. Celery is a great addition to smoothie and juice recipes.

- Carrots – PRAL -4.9

Carrots are another great alkaline food and they are also famous for improving eyesight due to their vitamin A content. Just a single cup of carrots has more than 300% of the recommended daily intake of beta-carotene, which is the antioxidant form of vitamin A. Beta-carotene also has the ability to protect against cancer and it helps your skin to look younger and brighter.

- Kiwi – PRAL -4.1

Kiwi is another delicious fruit that is highly alkalizing. It contains a plethora of minerals, vitamins, and antioxidants. While oranges have long been the kind of vitamin C, kiwi fruit contains almost five times the amount of vitamin C than an orange does. Kiwi also provides your body with fiber to help improve your digestion, and it contains potassium, which helps with muscle function.

- Tubers – PRAL -5.6

While you are working on trying to decrease the grains you eat, you might be asking what in the world can I eat to fill in this void. This answer is simple, tubers. Tubers are plants that develop starchy roots and are foods from ancient civilizations. They have been prized for their wonderful benefits. They are considered complex carbs, tubers give our bodies blood sugar. They provide stabilizing slow-burning energy. They are high in antioxidants, magnesium, potassium, vitamins C and A, phytochemicals, and fiber. Tubers can help lower the risk of heart disease, lowers the risk of cancer, and keeps your bones healthy. Tubers are a low-calorie option to be used in place of other starchy, grain-based carbs. Your best bet is cassava, yams, and sweet potatoes.

You don't have to feel guilty about your love for sweet potatoes fires. While they may be a starchy vegetable, sweet potatoes are amazingly alkalizing, and it provides your body with lots of minerals, vitamins, and fiber. Since sweet potatoes have a high fiber content, they don't have as much of an impact on your blood sugar levels, since the fiber content works to slow down the release of sugar to your bloodstream. Therefore, sweet potatoes are a great food to consume when you need some energy and some alkalinity.

Recipes

Breakfast

Hemp Seed and Carrot Muffins

Serves: 12

Cashew butter, 6 tbsp

Shredded carrot,

Unrefined whole cane sugar, .5 c.

Almond milk, 1 c.

Oat flour, 2 c.

Ground flaxseed, 1 tbsp

Water, 3 tbsp

Pinch of sea salt

Vanilla bean powder, pinch

Baking powder, 1 tbsp

Chopped kale, 1 tbsp

Hemp seeds, 2 tbsp

1. Start by placing your oven to 350.

2. Beat the flaxseed and water together to make the flax egg.

3. Pour this into a bigger bowl then combine within the salt, vanilla bean-flavored powder, baking powder, kale, hemp seeds, cashew butter, carrot, sugar, almond milk, and oat flour. Stir everything together until well combined.

4. Grease a 12-cup muffin tin and divide the batter between the cups. Bake for 20-25 minutes and enjoy.

Chia Seed and Strawberry Parfait

Serves: 2

Strawberry Mixture –

Brown rice syrup, 1-2 tsp

Chia seeds, 1 tsp

Diced strawberries, 1 c.

Oat Mixture –

Quick rolled oats, 1 c.

Vanilla bean powder, pinch

Brown rice syrup, 1 tbsp

Coconut milk, 1 c.

1. To make the strawberry mixture, stir together the brown rice syrup, chia seeds, and strawberries in a small bowl until well-mixed.

2. In a separate bowl, mix together the vanilla bean powder, brown rice syrup, coconut milk, and oats until well-mixed.

3. Place portion of the oats in the base of two small jars. Cover with a portion of the strawberry mixture. Repeat this with the remaining ingredients.

4. Put a cover on the jars and let them to refrigerate all night long.

5. The next morning, uncover and enjoy.

Pecan Pancakes

Serves: 5

Chopped pecans, .25 c.

Nutmeg, .25 tsp

Cinnamon, .5 tsp

Vanilla, 1 tsp

Melted butter, 2 tbsp

Unsweetened soy milk, .75 c.

Eggs, 2

Salt, .25 tsp

Baking powder, .25 tsp

Granular sugar substitute, 1 tbsp

Almond flour, .75 c.

Olive oil - cooking spray

1. Place the salt, sugar substitute, baking powder, and almond flour into a bowl and mix well.

2. In another bowl, put the vanilla, soy milk, butter, and eggs. Mix well to incorporate everything.

3. Place the egg mixture into the dried-up contents and mix well till well-blended.

4. Add nutmeg, pecans, and cinnamon. Stir for five minutes.

5. Place a twelve-inch cooking pan onto average hot temperature and sprinkle by using cookery spray.

6. Scoop one tablespoon of batter into the preheated skillet and spread out into a four-inch circle.

7. Place three more spoonfuls into the skillet and cook until bubbles have formed at the edges of the pancakes and the bottoms are browned.

8. Flip each one and cook another two minutes.

9. Repeat the process until all batter has been used.

10. Serve with syrup of choice.

Quinoa Breakfast

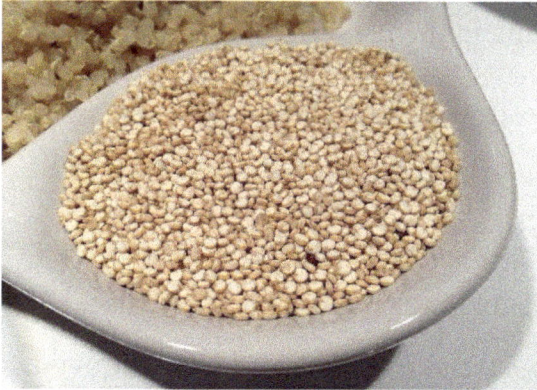

Serves: 4

Maple syrup, 3 tbsp

2-inch cinnamon stick

Water, 2 c.

Quinoa, 1 c.

Optional Toppings:

Yogurt

Chopped cashew, 2 tbsp

Whipped coconut cream, 3 tbsp

Lime juice, 1 tsp

Nutmeg, .25 tsp

Raisins, 2 tbsp

Strawberries, .5 c.

Raspberries, .5 c.

Blueberries, .5 c.

1. Put the quinoa into a strainer and rinse it under cold running water. Make sure there aren't any stones or anything in them.

2. Pour water into a saucepan. Add the quinoa and place saucepan on medium heat. Bring to a boil.

3. Add in the cinnamon stick, place a cover on the saucepan, lower hot temperature, also, boil gently quarter-hour till water has been ingested.

4. Take off hot temperature and fluff with a fork. Add maple syrup and any of the toppings listed above.

Oatmeal

Serves: 4

Salt

Steel-cut oats, 1.25 c.

Water, 3.75 c.

Optional Toppings:

Nuts

Dried fruits

Sliced banana

Diced mangoes

Mixed berries

Garam masala, 1 tsp

Lemon pepper, .25 tsp

Nutmeg, .25 tsp

Cinnamon, 1 tsp

1. Place a saucepan on medium and add water. Let the water boil.

2. Pour in the oats along with a dash of salt and lower the heat to a simmer.

3. Let simmer 25 minutes, stirring constantly.

4. Once all the water has been absorbed, add in any of the toppings listed above if you want to add in any flavor. If you want it creamier, add in a tablespoon of coconut milk.

Baked Grapefruit

Serves: 1

Unsweetened grated coconut, 2 tbsp

Halved grapefruit, 1

1. You need to warm your oven to 350.

2. Take some foil and line a baking sheet with it.

3. Place the halved grapefruit cut side up on the foil. Top each with one tablespoon of coconut.

4. Put into broiler and prepare quarter-hour or till coconut is tanned.

5. Carefully remove from oven and enjoy.

Almond Pancakes

Serves: 4

Coconut oil, 3 tbsp

Almond milk, 1 c.

Baking powder, 1 tsp

Arrowroot powder, 2 tbsp

Almond flour, 1 c.

1. Place each of the dry fixings in a dish and whip to mix.

2. Add two tablespoons of coconut oil together with almond milk to the dry fixings and blend well till everything is all around blended.

3. Place a skillet on medium and put one teaspoon coconut in it to melt. Swirl it around in the skillet to coat.

4. Pour one ladle of batter into the skillet and using the bottom of the ladle to smooth out pancake.

5. Cook for three minutes until edges are bubbly and brown.

6. Flip pancake and cook another three minutes until cooked through.

7. Continue cooking pancakes until all batter is used.

Amaranth Porridge

Serves: 2

Cinnamon, 1 tbsp

Coconut oil, 2 tbsp

Amaranth, 1 c.

Alkaline water, 2 c.

Almond milk, 2 c.

1. Flow the water together with the milk into a pot. Place on medium hot temperature and allow to boil.

2. Stir in amaranth and turn down the hot temperature to a low level. Stew for half an hour mixing every now and then.

3. Take off hot temperature, add in copra oil and cinnamon, stir well, serve warm.

Banana Porridge

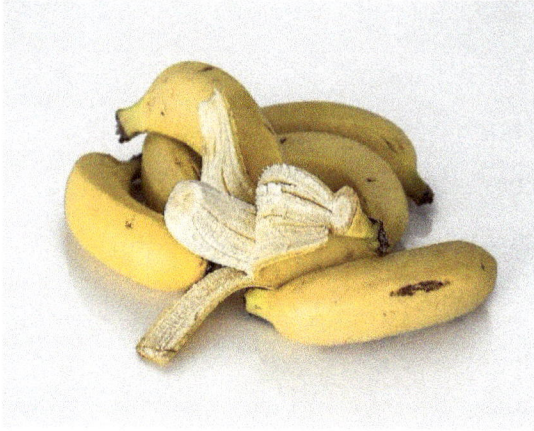

Serves: 2

Chopped almonds, .25 c.

Liquid stevia, 3 drops

Barley, .5 c.

Sliced banana, 1

Unsweetened almond milk, 1 c.

1. Mix the stevia, one half cup almond milk, and barley in a bowl.

2. Place in the refrigerator, covered for six hours.

3. Take out of the refrigerator and mix in the remaining milk. Pour into a saucepan and place on medium. Allow mixture to cook for five minutes.

Zucchini Muffins

Serves: 16

Salt

Cinnamon, 1 tsp

Baking powder, 1 tbsp

Almond flour, 2 c.

Vanilla extract, 1 tsp

Almond milk, .5 c.

Grated zucchinis, 2

Overripe bananas, 3

Almond butter, .25 c.

Alkaline water, 3 tbsp

Ground flaxseed, 1 tbsp

Optional Ingredients:

Chopped walnuts, .25 c.

Chocolate chips, .25 c.

1. You need to warm your kitchen appliance to 375 degrees. Sprinkle a cupcake tin by using cookery spray.

2. Place the water and flaxseed in a bowl.

3. Mash the bananas in a pot and put in altogether the leftover contents. Blend nicely.

4. Separate concoction evenly in a cupcake tin.

5. Place into the oven for 25 minutes.

Vegetable Tofu Scramble

Serves: 4

Salt

Chopped basil, 2 tbsp

Chopped firm tofu, 3 c.

Diced peppers (red, bell), 2 pcs.

Olive oil, 1 tablespoon

Turmeric

Chopped cherry tomatoes, 2 c.

Chopped onions, 2

Cayenne

1. Place a greased skillet on medium and warm the pan.

2. Put on bell peppers together with onions, prepare for five minutes.

3. Put in tofu, cayenne, salt, and turmeric. Cook an additional eight minutes.

4. Garnish with basil.

Zucchini Pancakes

Serves: 8

Finely chopped scallions, .5 c.

Finely chopped jalapeno, 2

Olive oil, 2 tsp

Ground flax seeds, 4 tbsp

Salt

Grated zucchini, 6

Alkaline water, 12 tbsp

1. Place the flax seeds and water into a bowl and mix well. Sit to the side.

2. Place a large skillet on medium and warm oil. Add on pepper, salt, and zucchini. Cook three minutes and place zucchini in a bowl.

3. Add in flaxseed mixture and scallions and mix well.

4. Warm a griddle that has been sprayed with cooking spray. Pour some zucchini onto the preheated griddle and cook three minutes per side until golden.

5. Repeat until mixture is completely used up.

Pumpkin Quinoa

Serves: 2

Chia seeds, 2 teaspoons

Pumpkin pie spice, 1 teaspoon

Pumpkin puree, .25 c.

Mashed banana, 1

Unsweetened almond milk, 1 c.

Cooked quinoa, 1 c.

1. Put all ingredients into a container.

2. Make sure the lid is sealed and shake well to combine.

3. Place in the refrigerator overnight.

4. When ready to eat, take out of the fridge and enjoy.

Avocado Toast

Serves: 4

Dulse flakes, sliced radish, sliced red onion, for topping – optional

Sea salt, .5 tsp

Fresh cilantro leaves, 1 tbsp

Chopped onion, 1 tbsp

Garlic, 2 cloves

Jalapeno

Avocado, 2

Unpeeled sweet potato, sliced into 4 thick lengthwise slices

1. Lay each of the slices of potato in a toaster slot and toast them for four cycles, or until they are cooked through. You can also toast them in the oven if you don't have a regular toaster. You want them to get tender enough to be pierced easily with a fork. Carefully place the cooked "toast" on plates.

2. Since the sweet potato toast cooks, add the salt, cilantro, onion, garlic, jalapeno, and avocado in an exceedingly electric kitchen appliance and blend till it becomes creamy and smooth. Adjust the amount of salt you use as needed.

3. Divide the avocado spread over the top each of the sweet potato toast slices. Top each with your desired toppings of choice. Enjoy.

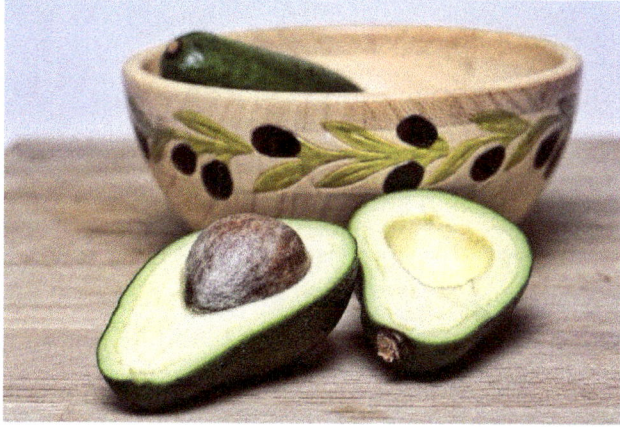

Frozen Banana Breakfast Bowl

Serves: 1

Chia seeds, hemp seeds, unsweetened coconut flakes, for topping – optional

Pumpkin seed protein powder, 4 tbsp

Bananas, 2

1. Peel and then slice the bananas. Place thin in a freezer-safe container and freeze them overnight.

2. The next morning, add the bananas to a food processor and mix until they reach a creamy and smooth consistency, much like soft-serve ice cream.

3. Process the pumpkin protein powder through the bananas until just combined.

4. Pour into a serving dish and top with your desired toppings if you so choose to and enjoy.

Chia Seed and Blueberry Cobbler

Serves: 4

Blueberry Mixture –

Chia seeds, 1 tbsp

Unrefined whole cane sugar, 2 tbsp

Blueberries, 2 c.

Topping –

Almond flour, .5 c.

Sea salt, .25 teaspoon

Vanilla bean powder, 1 teaspoon

A mixture of Sodium Bicarbonate and cream of tartar, 1.5 teaspoon

Unrefined whole cane sugar, 2 tablespoons

Melted coconut oil, 2 tablespoons

Coconut milk, 4 tablespoons

Oat flour, .5 c.

1. Start by placing your oven to 350.

2. To get the blueberries ready, mix the chia seeds, sugar, and blueberries together. Place the blueberry mixture into the bottom of four 4-ounce ovenproof ramekins.

3. To fix the topping, mix together the salt, vanilla bean powder, baking powder, sugar, coconut oil, coconut milk, oat flour, and almond flour.

4. Divide the topping over the blueberries in the four ramekins. You can either leave the topping as dollops, or you can spread them out evenly over the blueberry mixture to create a full crust.

5. Bake the cobblers for 45 minutes, or until the topping has turned golden and everything is heated through. Enjoy.

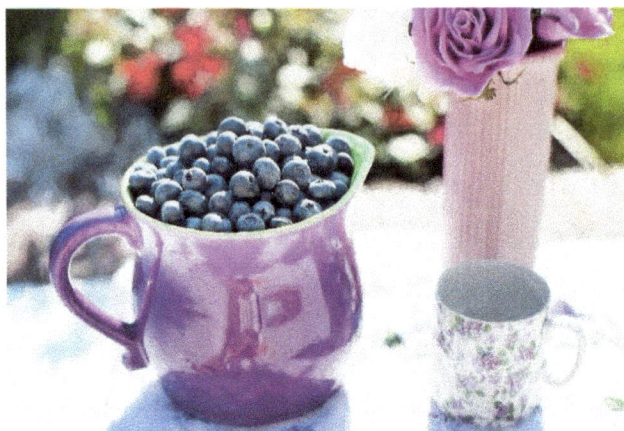

Quick and Easy Granola Bars

Serves: 6

Vanilla bean powder, .25 teaspoon

Cinnamon spice, .25 teaspoon

Seawater salt, .25 teaspoon

Coconut oil, 1 tablespoon

Brown rice syrup, 2 tablespoons

Almond butter, .5 c.

Quick rolled oats, 1 c.

1. Place some parchment into the bottom of a 9x5 inch loaf pan.

2. Add the vanilla bean powder, cinnamon, salt, coconut oil, brown rice syrup, almond butter, and oats to a food processor and mix until they are well-combined.

3. Run the concoction into the loaf frying pan as well as push it down into an even mixture, ensure that it's well-compressed. Refrigerate the bars for 15 to 20 minutes, or until they are completely firm.

4. Slice the granola into six bars and enjoy. Keep any leftovers in the refrigerator. At room temp, they will become soft.

Lunch

Roasted Artichoke Salad

Serves: 2

Paprika, pinch

Garlic powder, pinch

Pepper, pinch

Sea salt, pinch

Avocado oil, 1 tbsp

Drained artichoke hearts, 14 oz

Mixed salad greens, 2-4 c.

Dressing –

Pepper, pinch

Sea salt, pinch

Diced shallot

Brown rice sweetening, 1 tablespoon

Sesame pits, 1 tablespoon

Apple vinegar, 2 tablespoons

Avocado oil, 2 tbsp

1. Start by placing your oven to 425. Place some parchment on a baking sheet.

2. Slice the tips off of the artichokes and then slice the hearts in half. Rub them with some oil.

3. Mix together the paprika, garlic, pepper, and salt. Lay the artichokes on the baking sheet and sprinkle them with the seasoning mixture. Toss everything to coat.

4. Roast them for 30 minutes, tossing again halfway through the cooking time.

5. As the artichokes roast, beat together the pepper, salt, shallot, brown rice syrup, sesame seeds, vinegar, and avocado oil. Make sure everything is well mixed. Adjust any of the flavors as you need.

6. To assemble the salad, toss the mixed salad greens with the artichokes and then drizzle on the dressing. Divide into two plates and enjoy.

Sunchoke Hash

Serves: 4

Sliced scallion

EVOO

Pepper

Salt

Thinly sliced Brussels sprouts, 6

Sliced sunchokes, 4

1. Pour some cold water into a bowl.

2. Place the sliced sunchokes into the water and let them sit.

3. Rinse thoroughly and dry using paper towels.

4. Place a pan on medium and warm up some EVOO.

5. Add the sunchokes and Brussels sprouts. Cook for four minutes.

6. Sprinkle with pepper and salt.

7. Serve with a drizzle of olive oil and sprinkle on the sliced scallions.

Vegetable Fritters

Serves: 2

Cooking spray

Water, .25 c.

Garlic powder, .5 tsp

Salt, 1 tsp

Almond flour, .25 c.

Scallions, 4

Grated onion, .5

Chopped yellow squash, 1

Peeled and chopped carrot, 1

Chopped zucchini, 1

1. Place the scallion, almond flour, yellow squash, zucchini, carrot, garlic powder, and salt into a food processor.

2. Pulse until everything is thoroughly blended.

3. Add just enough water to make sure mixture is moist and thick.

4. Place an oversized pan on standard heat and sprinkle by using preparation spray.

5. When the oil is heated, use an ice cream scoop and add put mixture into skillet. Cook for three minutes each side.

6. Use back of ice cream scoop to spread the mixture around.

Mint Lime Salad

Serves: 4

Lemon juice, 2 tbsp

Chopped mint, 2 tbsp

Strawberries, .25 c.

Diced Peaches, .25 c.

Tangerine segments, .25 c.

Bite-size cantaloupe pieces, .25 c.

Bite-size honeydew pieces, .25 c.

Bite-size watermelon pieces, .25 c.

Diced apple, .25 c.

Grapes, .25 c.

1. Put all fruits into a bowl. Add in mint and lemon juice.

2. Mix well and cover.

3. Place in the refrigerator and chill overnight.

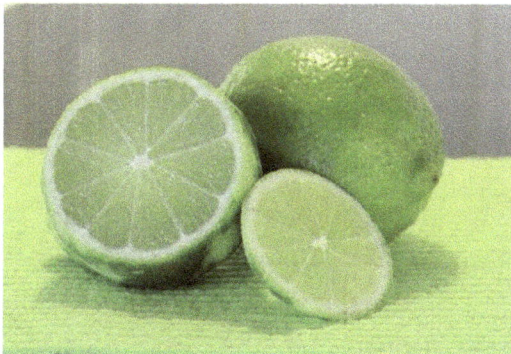

Zucchini Salad

Serves: 2

Fresh herbs of choice, 1 tsp

Pepper

Salt

EVOO, 2 tbsp

Juice of .5 lemon

Minced garlic, 1 clove

Sliced onion, 1

Diced tomato, 2

Red bell pepper, 1

Sliced zucchini, 1

4. Wash all vegetables and set to the side.

5. Cut the ends off the zucchini. Cut in half lengthwise and then slice into half-moons.

6. Dice the tomatoes.

7. Cut the bell pepper in half, clean out the ribs and seeds and slice each half.

8. Cut the top and bottom off the onion and remove outer peel. Thinly slice into rings.

9. Add all the prepared vegetables into a bowl.

10. In a separate bowl add pepper, salt, herbs, olive oil, garlic, and lemon juice. Mix well to combine.

11. Pour over vegetables and toss to coat.

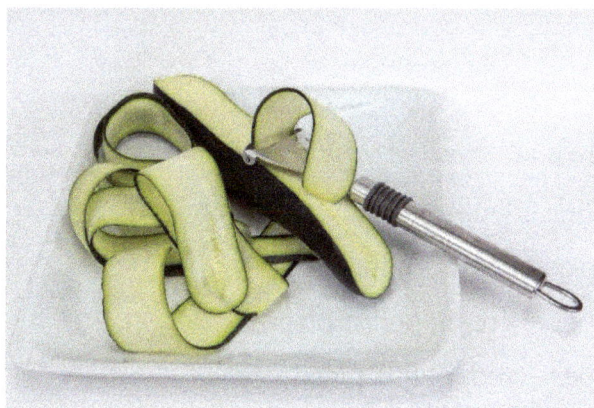

Stir Fried Tofu

Serves: 4

Fresh herbs

Ginger, .25 tbsp

Curry powder, .5 tbsp

Pepper

Salt

EVOO, 2 tbsp

Coconut milk, 1.5 c.

Chopped green beans, .5 lb.

Diced pepper – green, bell, 1 piece

Diced pepper – red, bell, 1 piece

Diced tomatoes, 3

Chopped zucchinis, 3

Diced firm tofu, 1 lb.

1. Place a saucepan on medium, warm oil. Add in tofu and cook about three minutes.

2. Add in zucchini, beans, and bell peppers. Stir fry for an additional three minutes.

3. Add tomatoes and coconut milk and stir well. Let it simmer for a little more time.

4. Season with herbs, curry powder, pepper, salt, and ginger.

5. Serve with wild rice.

Potato Pumpkin Patties

Serves: 2

EVOO

Pepper

Salt

Chopped parsley, 3 tbsp

Water, 4 tbsp

Soy flour, 2.5 oz

Potatoes, 1 lb.

Pumpkin, 1 lb.

1. Peel the potatoes and pumpkin. Cut them into large chunks.

2. Place into a food processor and process until small pieces but not mush.

3. Add the water and soy flour to a bowl. Mix well.

4. Take the pumpkin and potato out of the food processor and place them into a different bowl.

5. Pour on the flour mixture and mix well.

6. Season with pepper, parsley, and salt.

7. Place a skillet on medium and warm up some EVOO.

8. Turn the potato and pumpkin mixture into patties. Place prepared patties into the skillet and fry for three minutes per side.

Italian Stir-Fry

Serves: 2

Water, .5 c

Pepper

Curry powder, .5 teaspoon

Oregano plant, 1 teaspoon

Parsley, one tablespoon

Sodium Chloride, 1 teaspoon

Grated cheddar, 1 tbsp

EVOO, 2 tbsp

Diced tomatoes, 2

Slivered zucchini, 1

Diced onion, 2

Slivered leeks, 2

1. Take a skillet and place on medium warm up the olive oil.

2. Put the onions into the skillet and cook until soft.

3. Add zucchini and cook another four minutes. Pour water into the skillet and place a lid on it.

4. Lower heat and simmer for ten minutes.

5. Carefully remove the lid and add tomatoes. Season with curry powder and pepper. Replace lid and cook an additional ten minutes.

6. When cooked through, taste and adjust seasonings if needed.

7. Sprinkle with cheese and serve with bread if your diet allows it.

Southern Salad

Serves: 4

Salsa, .5 c.

Cilantro, .5 c.

Chopped almonds, .25 c.

Diced avocado, 1

Halved cherry tomatoes, 1 c.

Sprouted black beans, .5 c.

Romaine lettuce, 5 c.

1. Put each of the contents into an oversized bowl then throw nicely.

2. Divide into salad bowls and serve.

Roasted Vegetables

Serves: 4

Salt

Alliaceous (garlic) powder, 1 tablespoon

Coconut oil, 1 tablespoon

Pepper – chopped, bell – yellow, one

Pepper – chopped, bell - red, one

Chopped carrot, one

Trimmed asparagus, .5 bunch

Cherry tomatoes, 1 pint

Halved mushrooms, .5 c.

1. You need to warm your oven to 425.

2. Place the carrot, bell peppers, tomatoes, mushrooms, and asparagus into a large bowl.

3. In another basin, put in the garlic powder, Sodium Chloride, together with coconut milk. Blend nicely.

4. Run over the vegetables and toss to coat.

5. Pour vegetables onto a cooking film then place in the stove for 15 minutes till veggies are tender.

6. Divide onto four plates and enjoy.

Pad Thai Salad

Serves: 2

Salt, .5 tsp

Stevia, 1 packet

Tamarind paste, 1 tsp

Minced garlic, 1 clove

Juice of one lime

Chopped almonds, 2 tbsp

Chopped scallions, 1

Stripped zucchini, 1

Thinly sliced carrot, 2

Bean sprouts, 1 c.

Iceberg lettuce, 4 c.

1. Place the almonds, bean sprouts, zucchini, carrots, and lettuce into a large bowl.

2. Place the salt, stevia, lime juice, tamarind paste, and garlic into a small food processor. Process until well blended.

3. Pour dressing over the vegetables and toss to coat.

4. Evenly divide into serving bowls.

Cucumber Salad

Serves: 4

Pepper

Salt

Sesame seed oil, 3 tbsp

Minced garlic, 4 cloves

Cucumber, 1 lb.

1. Place the pepper, salt, sesame seed oil, and garlic to a bowl. Whisk well to combine.

2. Wash cucumbers and cut the ends off. Cut them in half lengthwise and then slice into half-moons.

3. Add to dressing mixture to the cucumbers and toss well to coat.

4. Place in the refrigerator for ten minutes. Enjoy.

Red Lentil Pasta Salad

Serves: 4

For the Dressing and Pasta –

Pepper, .25 tsp

Sea salt, .25 tsp

Dried oregano, 1 tsp

Juice - Lemon, one tablespoon

Apple vinegar, two tablespoons

Avocado - oil, .25 c.

Red lentil pasta, 2 c.

Veggies –

Crushed garlic, 2 cloves

Sliced summer squash, .5

Sliced zucchini, .5

Diced red onion, .33 c.

Chopped pepper – orange, bell, 1 c.

Chopped asparagus stalks, 6

Avocado oil, 1 tbsp

1. Cook the pasta following the directions on the package.

2. As the pasta is cooking, whisk the pepper, salt, oregano, lemon juice, vinegar, and avocado oil together until well combined. Adjust any of the seasonings that you need to.

3. For the veggies, warm the oil in an exceedingly frying pan then cook the garlic bulb, squash, zucchini, onion, bell pepper, and asparagus. Cook for two to three minutes, or until they are soft.

4. Add the pasta, veggies, and dressing in a bowl and toss everything together. Divide into four plates and enjoy.

Peach Salsa Salad

Serves: 2

Dressing –

Pinch sea salt

Lemon juice, 1 tsp

Water, .25 c

Brown rice syrup, 3 to 4 tbsp

Tahini, 4 tbsp

Salsa –

Diced jalapeno, .5

Chopped purple onion, one tablespoon

Diced coriander, one tablespoon

Chopped pepper – red, bell, .25 c.

Cubed and pitted peach

Assembling –

Mixed salad greens – 3 c

1. For the dressing, whisk together the salt, lemon juice, water, brown rice syrup, and tahini until combined. Adjust any of the seasonings that you need to.

2. Throw each of the condiment ingredients along inside another container.

3. To make the salad, place the salad greens on two plates and top with the salsa. Drizzle on the dressing and enjoy.

Pineapple Salad

Serves: 1

Dressing –

Chopped cilantro, .5 c.

Chopped scallions, .5 c.

Lime juice, 2 tbsp

Water, .25 c.

Avocado oil, .25 c.

Sea salt, .5 tsp

Garlic, 2 cloves

Assembling –

Dulse flakes

Chopped purple cabbage, 1 c.

Cubed pineapple, .5 c.

Mixed salad greens, 2 c.

1. Put each of the dressing contents to your liquidizer then blend till nicely combined. Adjust any of the seasonings that you need to.

2. To make your salad, add the salad green to a bowl and top with the dulse flakes, purple cabbage, and pineapple. Drizzle on the dressing and toss together. Enjoy.

Sweet Potato Salad with Jalapeno Dressing

Serves: 2

Sweet Potatoes –

Sea salt, .25 tsp

Paprika, 1 tsp

Crushed garlic, 2 cloves

Avocado oil, 2 tbsp

Peeled and cubed sweet potatoes, 3

Dressing –

Water, 1 c.

Sea salt, .5 tsp

Lime juice, 2 tbsp

Jalapeno

Cilantro leaves, .25 c.

Raw cashews, 1 c.

Assembling –

Mixed salad greens, 2 c.

1. Start by placing your kitchen appliance to three hundred and fifty degrees. Put some parchment on a cooking film.

2. Toss the cubed sweet potatoes in the salt, paprika, garlic, and avocado oil. Make sure that the potatoes are well-coated.

3. Lay the sweet potatoes out on the baking sheet and cook them for 25 minutes, or until they become soft.

4. As the potatoes cook, add the salt, lime juice, jalapeno, cilantro, cashews, and water to a high-speed blender and mix until smooth.

5. To make the salad, divide the salad greens into two plates and top with the cooked sweet potatoes. Top with the dressing and toss everything together.

Asparagus Salad with Lemon Dressing

Serves: 2

Salad –

Pepper, .25 tsp

Sea salt, .5 tsp

Crushed garlic, 3 cloves

Diced onion, .5 c.

Diced asparagus stalks, 24

Avocado oil, 1 tsp

Dressing –

Pepper

Sea salt, .25 tsp

Lemon juice, 2 tbsp

Water, .5 c.

Raw cashews, .5 c.

Assembling –

Mixed salad greens, 2 c.

1. For the asparagus, warm the oil in a massive frying pan and put in the pepper, salt, garlic, onion bulb, then the asparagus. Prepare for five until seven minutes, or till the onion has become soft.

2. To make the dressing, add half of the cooked asparagus mixture to a blender along with the pepper, salt, lemon

juice, water, and cashews. Blend up they are smooth and creamy.

3. To make your salad, divide the mixed greens between two plates and top with the rest of the cooked asparagus. Top with the dressing and enjoy.

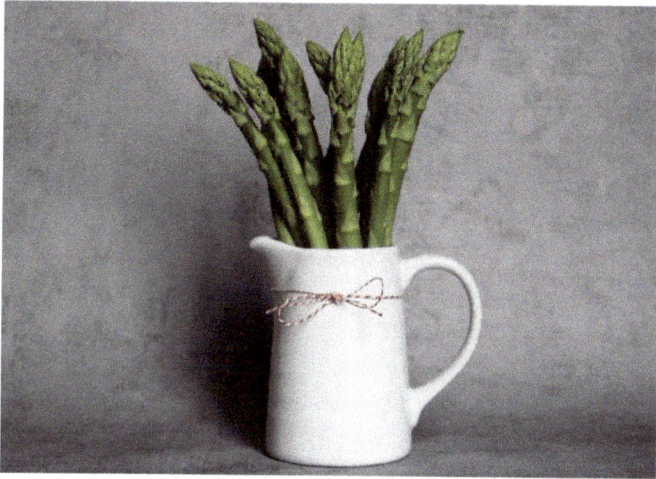

Dinner

Beefless Stew

Serves: 4

Dried oregano, 1 tsp

Diced celery, 2 stalks

Cubed large potato

Sliced carrot, 3 c.

Water, 2 c.

Vegetable broth, 3 c.

Pepper, one teaspoon

Seawater salt, one teaspoon

Mashed garlic, 2 bulbs

Diced onion, 1 c.

Avocado oil, 1 tbsp

Bay leaf

1. Heat up the avocado oil in an exceeding pot. Put in pepper, salt, garlic cloves, then onion bulbs. Cook everything for two to three minutes, or until the onion becomes soft.

2. Mix in the bay leaf, oregano, celery, potato, carrot, water, and broth. Allow this to come up to a simmer so that lower the heat down then prepare for 30-45 minutes, or until the carrots and potatoes become soft.

3. Taste and adjust the seasonings that you need to. If it is too thick, you can add some more water or broth.

4. Divide into four bowls and enjoy.

Emmenthal Soup

Serves: 2

Cayenne

Nutmeg

Pumpkin seeds, 1 tbsp

Chopped chives, 2 tbsp

Cubed Emmenthal cheese, 3 tbsp

Vegetable broth, 2 c.

Cubed potato, 1

Cauliflower pieces, 2 c.

1. Place the potato and cauliflower into a saucepan with the vegetable broth just until tender.

2. Place into a blender and puree.

3. Add in spices and adjust to taste.

4. Ladle into bowls, add in chives and cheese and stir well.

5. Garnish with pumpkin seeds. Enjoy.

Broccoli "Spaghetti"

Serves: 2

Pepper

Salt

Vegetable broth, 1 teaspoon

Oregano plant, 1 teaspoon

Juice - Lemon, 1 tablespoon

Sliced carrots, 3

Diced tomatoes, 3

Broccoli cut into floret, 1 head

Sliced pepper – red – bell, one

Sliced onion bulb, one

Diced garlic bulbs, two cloves

EVOO, 4 tbsp

Buckwheat pasta, 1 lb.

1. Place a pot of water on medium and add salt. Allow to boil and add in pasta. Prepare per box instructions. Empty out.

2. Place the broccoli into a different bowl and canopy with h2O. Prepare for five minutes.

3. Put a pan on normal heat and put in two tablespoons of olive oil into the skillet and warm. Put the bulbs, garlic, and onion then prepare till soft and scented. Remove from skillet then set to the side.

4. Add two more tablespoons of olive oil to the skillet and add carrots. Cook for five minutes, next put sweet pepper then prepare for another five minutes, now put in tomatoes then prepare for two minutes.

5. Completely drain the broccoli and add into the skillet with the rest of the vegetables. Put the onions and garlic back into the skillet.

6. Add vegetable broth, oregano, and lemon juice. Add some pepper and salt, taste and adjust seasonings if needed. Stir well to combine.

7. Place the cooked pasta onto a serving platter. Pour over vegetable mixture and toss to combine.

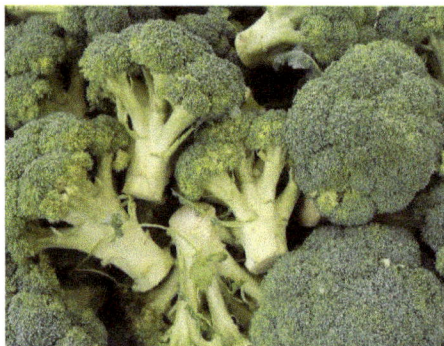

Indian Lentil Curry

Serves: 4 to 6

Lime juice

Chopped cilantro

Salt

EVOO, 1 tbsp

Diced tomatoes, 2

Sliced onion, 1

Minced garlic, 1 clove

Grated ginger, 1 inch

Turmeric, .5 tsp

Cumin seeds, .5 tsp

Chopped green chilies, 2

Fine red lentils, 1 c.

1. Place lentils into a bowl, cover with water and let sit for six hours.

2. After six hours, drain the lentils completely.

3. Place a basin on normal warmth. Put in the lentils then cover with fresh water. Allow to boil. Add in turmeric. Lower heat and simmer until lentils are cooked to your doneness.

4. Pull out from the pot then to a basin. Put these to side.

5. In another pan on medium, warm up olive oil. Add turmeric, cumin, ginger, and onions. Cook until onions are soft and ginger and fragrant.

6. Add chilies and tomatoes, and cook. Add salt and cook for five minutes.

7. Pour lentil into this mixture and bring back to a simmer. As shortly it begins to cook, remove it from the hot temperature. Squeeze in some lemon

8. Sprinkle with cilantro and serve with rice.

Vegetables with Wild Rice

Serves: 4

Salt

Basil

Cilantro

Juice of one lime

Chopped chili pepper, 1

Vegetable broth, .5 c.

Bean sprouts, 1 c.

Chopped carrots, 2 c.

Beans – green - diced, 1 c.

Broccoli, cleaved, 1 c.

Pak Choi, 1 c.

Wild rice, 1 c.

1. Place all the chopped vegetables into a pan and add vegetable broth.

2. Steam fry the vegetables until they are cooked through but still crunchy.

3. Using a mortar and pestle grind up the chili, basil, and cilantro until it forms a paste. Add in lime juice and mix well.

4. Place the rice onto a serving platter. Add the vegetables on top and drizzle with dressing.

Tangy Lentil Soup

Serves: 4

Salt

Turmeric, .25 tsp

Minced garlic, 3 cloves

Grated ginger, 1.5-inch piece

Chopped tomato, 1

Chopped Serrano Chile pepper, 1

Rinsed red lentils, 2 c.

Topping:

Coconut yogurt, .25 c.

1. Place the lentils in a colander and place under running water. Rinse until free from dirt and stones.

2. Pour rinsed lentils into a pot. Add enough water to cover lentils. Place the pot over medium heat and allow to boil.

3. Lower heat and simmer for ten minutes.

4. Put in the leftover contents then mix properly to blend.

5. Still, cook until lentils are soft.

6. Garnish with a spoonful of coconut yogurt.

Mushroom Leek Soup

Serves: 4

Sherry vinegar, 1.5 tbsp

Almond milk, .5 c.

Coconut cream, .66 c.

Vegetable broth, 3 c.

Chopped dill, 1 tbsp

Pepper

Salt

Almond flour, 5 tbsp

Cleaned, sliced mushrooms, 7 c.

Minced garlic, 3 cloves

Chopped leeks, 2.75 c.

Vegetable oil, 3 tbsp

1. Place a Dutch oven on medium and warm the oil. Add in the leeks together with garlic bulb then prepare till soft.

2. Put in the mushrooms, stir and cook an additional 10 minutes.

3. Add salt, dill, pepper, and flour. Stir well, until combined.

4. Put in soup and cause it to simmer. Lessen heat and put in rest of the ingredients. Stir well. Cook an additional ten minutes.

5. Serve warm with almond flour bread.

Fresh Veggie Pizza

Serves: 4

Crust –

Garlic bulb flavored powder, 0.5 teaspoon

Seawater salt, 0.5 teaspoon

Coconut oil, 3 tbsp

Almond flour, 1.25 c.

Tahini-Bee Spread –

Pepper, pinch

Sea salt, pinch

Garlic, 2 cloves

Juice - Lemon, one tablespoon

Avocado oil, one tablespoon

Middle eastern paste, one tablespoon

Peeled and cubed beets, 2

1. Start by placing your oven to 375. Place some parchment on a sheet tray.

2. Stir together the salt, garlic powder, coconut oil, and almond flour.

3. Place this on the sheet tray and squeeze into the shape of a ball. Place another piece of parchment on top and roll out the dough into 7x7 square. Bake for 14 minutes, or until it starts to brown.

4. As the crust bakes, add the pepper, salt, garlic, lemon juice, avocado oil, tahini, and beets to a food processor. Mix until it becomes creamy.

5. To make your pizza, spread the crust with beet sauces and then top with your favorite alkaline friendly veggies. Slice into four and enjoy.

Spicy Lentil Burgers

Serves: 4

Avocado oil, 1 tbsp

Coconut flour, 1 tbsp

Crushed garlic, 2 cloves

Diced jalapeno

Chopped cilantro, .5 c.

Diced onion, .5 c.

Pepper, .5 tsp

Sea salt, .5 tsp

Almond flour, .5 c.

Dry lentils, .5 c.

1. Cook the lentils following the directions on the package and set them to the side to cool off.

2. Mix together the garlic, jalapeno, cilantro, onion, pepper, salt, almond flour, and lentils until everything is well combined.

3. Add half of the lentil mixture to a food processor and process until it reaches a paste-like consistency.

4. Pour this back into the bowl with the rest of the lentil mixture and stir everything together. The mixture will be very moist. Stir in the coconut flour to help get rid of the moisture and to help them hold together.

5. Divide the mixture into fourths. Squeeze one-fourth of the mixture in your hands to flatten it out into a burger shape. Do this for the three remaining sections.

6. Warm up the oil in an exceedingly massive pot and put in the burgers. Prepare the burgers on 4 to 6 minutes on both sides, or until they have turned golden. When you flip them, do so carefully so that they don't fall apart. Enjoy.

Roasted Cauliflower Wraps

Serves: 2

Cauliflower –

Pepper, .25 tsp

Sea salt, .25 tsp

Garlic powder, .5 tsp

Nutritional yeast, .25 c.

Almond flour, .25 c.

Avocado oil, 1 tbsp

Bite-size cauliflower florets, 2 c.

Sauce –

Sea salt

Apple cider vinegar, 2 tbsp

Garlic, 2 cloves

Habanero pepper

Cubed mango, 1 c.

Assembling –

Collard greens, 2 leaves

Mixed salad greens, 1 c.

1. Start by placing your kitchen appliance to three hundred and fifty degrees then put a few papers on a cooking film.

2. To prepare your cauliflower, toss the cauliflower in the avocado oil and make sure they are evenly coated.

3. Into a container, combine along the all the seasonings: pepper, salt, garlic powder, healthy fungus, together with the almond flour.

4. Sprinkle the breading over the cauliflower and toss everything together making sure that the cauliflower is well-coated. Spread across the cooking film.

5. Cook it on about thirty up to thirty-five minutes, either that or till the cauliflower is soft.

6. As the cauliflower bakes, add the salt, vinegar, garlic, habanero, and mango to your blender and mix until well-combined. Make sure that you use some gloves or wash your hands really well when it comes to handling the habanero.

7. To assemble, divide the mixed salad greens between the collard leaves, top with the cauliflower and drizzle on the sauce. Wrap everything up like a burrito and enjoy.

Sliced Sweet Potato with Artichoke and Pepper Spread

Serves: 4

Pepper, .25 tsp

Salt, .5 tsp

Avocado oil, 6 tsp – divided

Quartered red bell pepper

Unpeeled sweet potatoes, 2 sliced into 4 lengthwise slices

Garlic, 2 cloves

Artichoke hearts, 14 oz can

1. Start by placing the oven to 350. Place some parchment on a sheet tray and set to the side.

2. Lay the bell pepper and sweet potato on the sheet tray and top them with two teaspoons of avocado oil, a pinch of pepper, and a pinch of salt.

3. Bake them for 30 minutes. Turn it over and cook to an additional fifteen minutes.

4. Add the roasted red bell pepper to a food processor along with the garlic, artichoke hearts, pepper, salt, and the remaining avocado oil. Pulse until combined but still a little chunky. Adjust any seasonings that you need.

5. Top the slices of sweet potato with the spread and enjoy.

Scallop Onion and Potato Bake

Serves: 4

Cashew Cheese Sauce –

Sea salt, .5 tsp

Nutritional yeast, .5 c.

Almond milk, 1 c.

Raw cashews, 1 c.

Scallop Bake –

Chopped tarragon, 1 tbsp

Pepper, 1 teaspoon

Seawater salt, one teaspoon

Oil – Avocado, one tablespoon

Chopped tiny onion bulbs, 1.5

Thinly sliced new potatoes, 8

1. To make the cheese sauce, add the cashews to a bowl and cover with room temperature water. Allow them to soak for 15 to 20 minutes and then drain and rinse.

2. Blend together the cashews with the remaining cheese sauce ingredients until smooth and creamy. Set to the side until later.

3. Start by heating the oven to 375.

4. Combine the onions and potatoes together in a bowl with the avocado oil. Toss in the tarragon, pepper, and salt, making sure everything is well coated.

5. Using an 8-inch square baking dish, place in the potato and onion mixture in the dish. Try your best to arrange them in nice rows. This doesn't have to be perfect.

6. Bake everything for 45 minutes, or until the potatoes become soft

7. Take it out of the oven and top with the cheese sauce. Divide between four plates and enjoy. You can also slide this, and cook inside the kitchen appliance on about 5 minutes in order to heat the caseous sauce through before serving.

Spicy Cilantro and Coconut Soup

Serves: 2

Cilantro leaves, 2 tbsp

Jalapeno

Lime juice, 1 tbsp

Full-fat coconut milk, 13.5 oz can

Sea salt, .25 tsp

Crushed garlic, 3 cloves

Diced onion, .5 c.

Avocado oil, 2 tbsp

1. Add the avocado oil to a medium pan and heat. Add in the salt, garlic, and onion, cooking for three to five minutes, either that or till the onion bulbs get to be smooth.

2. Put in the onion mixture, cilantro, jalapeno, lime juice, and coconut milk to a blender and mix until it becomes creamy.

3. Pour into a bowl and enjoy.

Tarragon Soup

Serves: 2

Chopped fresh tarragon, 2 tbsp

Celery stalk

Raw cashews, .5 c.

Lemon juice, 1 tbsp

Full-fat coconut milk, 13.5 oz can

Pepper, .5 tsp – divided

Sea salt, .5 tsp – divided

Crushed garlic, 3 cloves

Diced onion, .5 c.

Avocado oil, 1 tbsp

1. Add the oil to a medium pan and warm it up. Put in all the seasonings: pepper, salt, garlic bulbs, together with onion bulbs then prepare approximately three to five minutes, or until the onions turn soft.

2. Using a high-speed blender, add the onion mixture, tarragon, celery, cashews, lemon juice, and coconut milk. Blend everything together until smooth. Taste and adjust the seasonings as you need to.

3. Divide into two bowls and enjoy. You can also add back into a pot and heat through before serving.

Asparagus and Artichoke Soup

Serves: 4

Stemmed and halved artichoke hearts, 1 can

Almond milk, 2 c.

Pepper, .5 tsp

Sea salt, .5 - .75 tsp

Vegetable broth, 2 c.

Diced asparagus, 8 stalks

Cubed potatoes, 1 c.

Crushed garlic, 2 cloves

Avocado oil, 1 tbsp

Diced onion, .5 c.

1. Add the garlic, avocado oil, and onion in a skillet and cook for a few minutes, either that or till the onion bulbs have smoothened and weakened.

2. Put in the cooked veggies to a pot and add in the pepper, salt, vegetable broth, asparagus, and potatoes. Stir everything together and let it come up to a simmer. Lower the hot temperature and boil gently on about eighteen up to twenty minutes, either that or till the potatoes have become soft. Add in some extra broth if you find that you need to so that the liquid stays about an inch over the veggies.

3. Set the pot away from the fire then let it chill.

4. Using a blender, mix up the cooled soup with the artichokes and almond milk until everything is well-combined and smooth. Adjust any of the seasonings that you need to. You can add extra broth or milk to thick it out if needed.

5. Pour back into the pot and let it warm over low until ready to serve.

Mint and Berry Soup

Serves: 1

Sweetener –

Water, .25 c – plus more if needed

Unrefined whole cane sugar, .25 c.

Soup –

Water, .5 c.

Mixed berries, 1 c.

Mint leaves, 8

Lemon juice, 1 tsp

1. Add the water and sugar to a small pot and cook, stirring constantly, until the sugar has dissolved. Allow this to cool.

2. Add the mint leaves, lemon juice, water, berries, and the cooled sugar mixture to a blender. Mix everything together until smooth.

3. Pour into a basin then put in the refrigerator till the broth is completely chilled. This will take about 20 minutes.

4. Enjoy.

Mushroom Soup

Serves: 2

Full-fat coconut milk, 13.5 oz can

Vegetable broth, 1 c.

Pepper, .5 tsp

Sea salt, .75 tsp

Crush garlic clove

Diced onion, 1 cup

Cut up cremini mushrooms, 1 cup

Cut up Chinese black mushrooms, one cup

Avocado oil, 1 tbsp

Coconut aminos, 1 tbsp

Dried thyme, .5 tsp

1. Warm up the grease in a very massive pan then put in all the seasonings: pepper, salt, garlic, onion bulb, and mushrooms. Boil and prepare everything along for a few minutes, either that or till the onions turn soft.

2. Mix in the coconut aminos, thyme, coconut milk, and vegetable broth. Lower the fire down then allow the broth to boil on approximately a quarter-hour. Mix the broth from time to time.

3. Taste and adjust any of the seasonings that you need to. Divide into two bowls and enjoy.

Potato Lentil Stew

Serves: 4

Chopped oregano sprigs, 2 sprigs

Diced celery stalk

Cubed and peeled potato, 1 c.

Sliced carrots, 2

Dry lentils, 1 c.

Spicy condiment / Pepper, one teaspoon

Seawater salt, one to 1.5 teaspoon

Mashed garlic bulbs, two buds

Diced onion, .5 c.

Avocado oil, 2 tbsp

Full-fat coconut milk, 13.5 oz can

Vegetable broth, 5 c – divided

Chopped tarragon, 2 sprigs

1. Using a big cooking utensil, warm the avocado grease together with putting in seasonings: pepper, salt, garlic bulbs, together with onion. Cook for three to five minutes, or until the onion has become soft.

2. Mix in the tarragon, oregano, celery, potato, carrots, lentils, and 2 ½ cups of the vegetable broth. Mix everything together.

3. Enable the casserole to return up to heat and then lower the fire down. Let this cook, stirring often. Add in extra

vegetable broth in half cup portions as needed to make sure that the lentils have enough liquid to cook. Let the stew cook for 20 to 25 minutes, or until the lentils and potatoes are soft.

4. Set the stew off the heat and mix in the coconut milk. Divide into four bowls and enjoy.

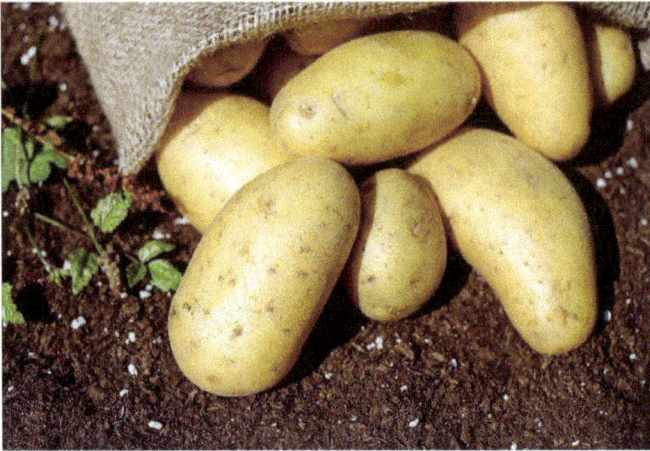

Snacks

Thanksgiving Pudding

Serves: 8

Coconut whipped cream

Cored, diced apples, .5 c.

Raisins, .5 c.

Salt

Cinnamon, 1 tsp

Unsweetened coconut milk, .5 c.

Unsweetened pumpkin puree, 1 can

1. You need to warm your oven to 350.

2. Place the nutmeg, salt, coconut milk, cinnamon, and pumpkin into kitchen appliance then pat till soft and even.

3. Put in the apples and raisins. Pulse a few times to combine.

4. Pour mixture into a 9-inch pie plate.

5. Place into the oven for one hour until the top is cracked just slightly.

6. Serve topped with whipped coconut cream.

Banana Muffins

Serves: 12

Split and deseeded vanilla bean, 1

Salt

Baking soda, 2 tsp

Melted coconut oil, .25 c.

Coconut flour, .5 c.

Creamy almond butter, .5 c.

Dates, 1 c.

Ripe bananas, 2.

Cooking spray

1. You need to warm your oven to 350. Place paper liners into a cupcake tin.

2. Place the dates and bananas into a food processor and process until well-blended. Add in vanilla bean seed, hydrogen carbonate, salt, coconut flour, copra oil, then almond butter. Process until batter forms.

3. Place batter into muffin tin until it is about 75 percent full.

4. Place into oven and bake eighteen minutes. The small cakes are finished once toothpick is placed in the center and turns out neat. Allow to cool slightly and enjoy.

Almost Crispy Rice Treatlets

Serves: 12

Brown rice cereal, 4 c.

Salt

Split and scraped vanilla bean, 1

Coconut oil, .25 c.

Brown rice syrup, .66 c.

Cooking spray

1. Using a nine-inch cooking platter, sprinkle it with some spray for cooking.

2. Put the saucepan on medium. Add in coconut oil and rice syrup and allow to boil for one minute.

3. Add salt and vanilla bean seed.

4. Place the rice cereal into a bowl. Pour syrup mixture over. Mix well until all cereal is coated.

5. Run through the readied pan. Put cooking spray into your hands then push the blended concoction to the pan to make an even layer.

6. Allow to sit for 45 minutes.

Fruit Crumble

Serves: 6

Salt

Softened coconut oil, one tablespoon

No-sugar grated coconut, .5 c.

Raw almonds, 1.5 c.

Split and scraped vanilla bean, 1

Stevia, 1 packet

Chopped summer fruits of choice like strawberries, plums, blueberries, etc., 2 c.

Cooking spray

1. You need to warm your oven to 350. Spray a nine-inch baking dish and set to the side.

2. Put a saucepan on medium heat. Add stevia, vanilla bean, and fruits. Stir well and allow to boil.

3. Add the coconut oil, salt, and almonds to a food processor. Pulse until crumbly mixture forms.

4. Place the fruit into a baking dish.

5. Top with almond mixture. Place in the oven for 15 minutes.

Pumpkin Crackers

Serves: 6

Alkaline water, 1.33 c.

Melted coconut oil, 3 tbsp

Salt

Psyllium husk powder, 1 tbsp

Sesame seeds, .33 c.

Flaxseed, .75 c.

Sunflower seeds, .75 c.

Pumpkin pie spice, 2 tbsp

Coconut flour, .33 c.

1. You need to warm your oven to 300. Take a cookie sheet and line it with paper.

2. Place every dry ingredient to a basin then stir well to combine.

3. Add in oil and water, and mix well. Allow the flour mixture to rest for 3 minutes.

4. Lay the flour mixture out onto prepared cookie sheet.

5. Place into the oven for 30 minutes. Lower temperature to 225 and continue to bake another 30 minutes.

6. Take out of the oven and crack the bread into pieces.

Apple Crisps

Serves: 4

Cinnamon, .5 tsp

White sugar, 1.5 tsp

Cored, thinly sliced apples, 2

1. You need to warm your kitchen appliance to two hundred twenty-five degrees. Lay out a cooking film with paper.

2. Combine cinnamon spice together with sugar together in a bowl.

3. Put apple slices into sugar mixture and toss to evenly coat.

4. Spread coated apples onto a prepared baking sheet. Place in oven for 45 minutes.

5. Take out of the oven and allow to cool slightly.

Peanut Butter Bars

Serves: 6

Vanilla, .5 tsp

Peanut butter, .5 c.

Swerve Sweetener, .25 c.

Almond butter, 2 oz

Almond flour, .75 c

1. Place all ingredients into a bowl and mix well until well-combined.

2. Place into a six-inch square pan. Press down firmly.

3. Place in the refrigerator for 30 minutes.

4. Take out of the refrigerator, evenly slice and serve.

Zucchini Chips

Serves: 4

Thinly sliced zucchini, 2

Pepper – red - gratings, three tablespoons

Pepper - regular

Onion flavored powder, one teaspoon

Garlic flavored powder, one teaspoon

Oil - vegetable, 1.66 cup

1. You need to warm your oven to 350.

2. Place the spices and oil into a bowl and mix well. Add in the zucchini and toss to evenly coat.

3. Place into a zip top bag and seal. Place in the refrigerator for ten minutes.

4. Take out of the refrigerator and spread sliced zucchini onto a greased baking sheet.

5. Place in the oven and bake 15 minutes.

6. Carefully remove from oven and let cool slightly.

Cashew Cream Stuffed Mushrooms

Serves: 6

Mushrooms –

Pinch pepper

Pinch sea salt

Avocado oil, 1.5 tsp

Stemmed cremini mushrooms, 12

Stuffing –

Sea salt, .25 teaspoon

Apple vinegar, one teaspoon

Juice - Lemon, 0.25 cup

Garlic bulbs, two cloves

Raw cashews, 1 c.

1. To prepare the mushrooms, rinse and dry the mushroom caps.

2. Add the oil to a medium-size pan. Place in the mushroom caps and sprinkle on some pepper and salt. Sauté them for a couple of minutes, or until soft. Get rid of the liquid that has accumulated in the pan.

3. For the stuffing, add the salt, vinegar, lemon juice, garlic, and cashews in a blender and mix until it creates a thick paste.

4. Spoon this into the mushroom caps and enjoy.

Garlic Breadsticks

Serves: 12

Breadsticks –

Pepper, 0.5 teaspoon

Seawater salt, 0.5 teaspoon

Oregano, chopped, one tablespoon

Oil - avocado, one tablespoon

Almond flour, 2 c.

Ground flaxseed, 1 tbsp

Water, 3 tbsp

Topping –

Avocado oil, 1 tbsp

Pepper

Sea salt

Chopped fresh oregano, 1 tbsp

Crushed garlic, 4 cloves

1. Start by placing your oven to 350. Place some parchment on a sheet tray.

2. To fix the breadstick, whisk the water and flaxseed together to make the flax egg.

3. Stir together the pepper, salt, oregano, avocado oil, almond flour, and flax egg until they come together and forms a dough.

4. Place the mixture on your prepared sheet tray and form it into a ball. Set an additional piece of paper above then utilize a kitchen utensil to flat the dough out into a 5x8 inch rectangle.

5. To make the topping, mix together the pepper, salt, oregano, garlic, avocado oil together. Pour the garlic oil over the dough and spread it out with the rear of a spoon.

6. Cook the breadsticks to about eighteen up to twenty minutes, either that or till it starts to brown.

7. Remove and slice into 12 pieces. Enjoy.

Tarragon Crackers

Serves: 5

Garlic powder, .25 tsp

Pepper, 0.5 teaspoon

Seawater salt, 0.5 teaspoon

Oil – avocado, one tablespoon

Daisy plant herb, one tablespoon

Almond flour, 2 c.

Ground flaxseed, 1 tablespoon

Water, 3 tbsp

1. Start by heating your kitchen appliance to three hundred and fifty degrees. Put some paper on a cooking film tray.

2. Beat the water and flaxseed together to make your flax egg.

3. Stir the garlic powder, pepper, salt, avocado oil, tarragon, and almond flour into the flax egg. Make sure everything comes together.

4. Place this on the baking sheet and then form it into a ball with your hands. Lay another sheet of parchment on top and roll the dough out to a quarter inch thickness.

5. With a knife or pizza cutter, slice the dough into 60 squares.

6. Bake them for 12 to 14 minutes. They should golden on top. Turn them over then cook them for an additional 2 minutes.

7. Cool the crackers and then enjoy.

Pear Nachos with Almond Butter

Serves: 1

Unsweetened shredded coconut flakes, 1 to 2 tsp

Hemp seeds, 1 to 2 tsp

Water, 1 to 2 tbsp – if needed

Cinnamon, pinch

Vanilla bean powder, pinch

Unrefined whole cane sugar, 2 to 3 tsp

Almond butter, 2 tbsp

Sliced and unpeeled pear

Slivered almonds, 1 tbsp

1. Lay the pear slices on a plate.

2. To fix the drizzle, add the cinnamon, vanilla bean powder, sugar, and almond butter to a bowl and mix together until everything is well-combined. Depending on how thick your almond butter is, you may need to add some water to help thin it out. You only want it to be thin enough so that you can drizzle it.

3. Drizzle the almond butter over the sliced pears. Top with some almonds, coconut flakes, and hemp seeds and enjoy. You can also dip the pear slices in any extra drizzle that you may have.

Chewy Seed and Nut Bars

Serves: 16

Vanilla bean powder, 1 tsp

Brown rice syrup, .25 c.

Unrefined whole cane sugar, .5 c.

Hemp seeds, .5 c.

Sesame seeds, .5 c.

Raw pumpkin seeds, .5 c.

Raw almonds, .75 c.

Raw cashews, .75 c.

Pinch sea salt

Cinnamon, 1 tsp

1. Start by placing your oven to 350 and lay some parchment into an 8-inch baking pan.

2. Mix together the hemp seeds, sesame seeds, pumpkin seeds, almonds, and cashews together.

3. Add the salt, cinnamon, vanilla bean powder, brown rice syrup, and sugar to a small pot and heat. Cook and stir until the sugar dissolves.

4. Quickly pour this over the seeds and nuts, and mix together until everything is well-coated.

5. Pour into the prepared pan and flatten out into an even layer using your hands. Bake for 18 to 20 minutes.

6. Allow this to cool completely for 30 to 45 minutes. Cut into 16 squares.

Cinnamon Cashews

Serves: 4

Raw cashews, 1.5 c.

Vanilla bean powder, .25 tsp

Cinnamon, .25 tsp

Unrefined whole cane sugar, .5 c.

Water, .5 c

1. Place some parchment on a sheet tray and set to the side.

2. Add the vanilla bean powder, cinnamon, sugar, and water in a small pot and cook until the sugar dissolves.

3. Add in the cashews and turn the heat up to med-high. Cook, stirring constantly, for four to six minutes. Do not step away from this. The sugary liquid is going to thicken and stick to the cashews. If you step away, it could end up hardening incorrectly.

4. Once the liquid has cooked away, set this off the heat and spread out on the sheet tray. You can move the cashews so that none of them are touching or you can let them form little clusters.

5. Let them cool and enjoy.

Coconut and Vanilla Truffles

Serves: 12

Sea salt

Vanilla bean fine grains, two teaspoons

Cashew nut butter, two tablespoons

Coconut flour, two tablespoons

Brown rice syrup, .25 c.

Coconut oil, .25 c.

Unsweetened coconut flakes, 2 c.

1. Add the vanilla bean powder, cashew butter, coconut flour, brown rice syrup, coconut oil, coconut flakes, and salt to a food processor and pulse until it creates a sticky mixture.

2. Let the mixture sit in the refrigerator for around 15 minutes, or until it has firmed up so that it will hold the shape of a ball.

3. Roll tablespoonfuls into balls and place in a lidded container. Keep them in the refrigerator until you want to serve them. They will end up becoming soft if you leave them at room temperature.

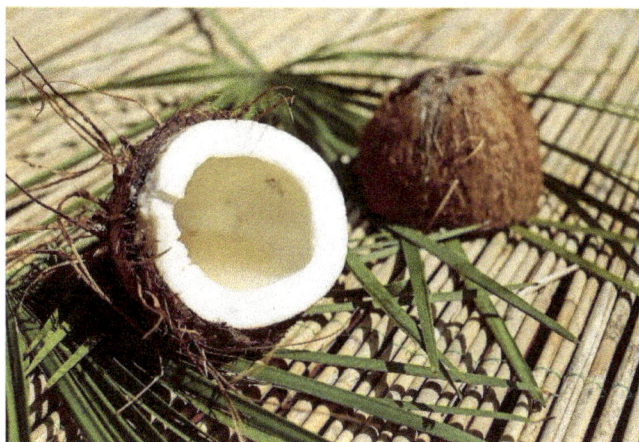

Cashew Butter Fudge

Serves: 16

Sesame seeds, hemp seeds, chia seeds, unsweetened shredded coconut flakes – optional toppings

Brown rice syrup, 2 tbsp

Melted coconut oil, .25 c.

Cashew butter, 1 c.

1. Stir the brown rice syrup, coconut oil, and cashew butter together until everything is well mixed.

2. Divide the fudge mixture between 16 mini muffin cups, filling them to about ¾ of the way full.

3. If you want, you can now top them with some sesame seeds, hemp seeds, chia seeds, or shredded coconut.

4. Place them in the freezer for a couple of hours to allow them to firm.

5. Keep them stored in the freezer until you want to enjoy one. They will become soft if they sit at room temperature.

Lime and Chia Seed Cookies

Serves: 12

Pinch sea salt

Brown rice syrup, .25 c.

Coconut flour, 2 tbsp

Chia seeds, two tablespoons

Juice - Lime, two tablespoons

Coconut oil, three up to four tablespoons – divided

Raw cashews, 2 c.

1. Start by placing your oven to 350 and place some parchment on a sheet pan.

2. Add two tablespoons of coconut oil and the cashews in a food processor and combine until you make cashew butter. This will take upwards of ten minutes and will go through several different steps. Stop every couple of minutes to scrape the sides down so that everything is blended evenly. You can add in more coconut oil if you need to, a tablespoon at a time, to make it creamier. Don't exceed four tablespoons.

3. Add the cashew butter to a bowl and add in the salt, brown rice syrup, coconut flour, chia seeds, and lime juice. Stir everything together.

4. Roll tablespoonfuls of the dough into balls and press them slightly into a disk shape. Place them on the sheet pan. Continue with the rest of the dough.

5. Bake the cookies for 12 minutes, making sure that they don't over-bake.

6. Let the cookies cool completely before taking them off the pan. They are going to be soft and crumbly when they first come out of the oven but will firm up as they cool. Enjoy.

Apple Crumble

Serves: 6

Apple Filling –

Juice from ¼ of a lemon

Cinnamon, .5 tsp

Brown rice syrup, 1 tbsp

Diced apple

Crumble –

Unrefined whole cane sugar, .5 c.

Almond flour, 2 c.

Ground flaxseed, 1 tbsp

Water, 3 tbsp

Pinch sea salt

Vanilla bean powder, pinch

Cinnamon, .5 tsp

Avocado oil, 1 tbsp

1. Start by setting your oven to 350. Place some parchment into a 9x5 inch loaf pan.

2. To prepare the apple filling, mix together the lemon juice, cinnamon, brown rice syrup, and apple and set to the side.

3. For the crumble, stir the water and flaxseed together to make the flax egg.

4. Mix together the salt, vanilla bean powder, cinnamon, avocado oil, sugar, almond flour, and flax egg till nicely blended.

5. Push down ½ of the crushed combination underneath the loaf pan.

6. Top the crumble with the apple filling and spread out evenly. Sprinkle the rest of the crumble over top of the apples.

7. Bake this for 20 to 25 minutes and enjoy.

Pumpkin Seed Cookies

Serves: 20

Sea salt, .25 tsp

Baking soda, .5 tsp

Brown rice syrup, 2 tbsp

Raw pumpkin seeds, .5 c.

Almond flour, .5 c.

Coconut oil, .5 c.

Raw cashews, 2 c.

1. Start by placing your oven to 350 and place some parchment on a sheet pan.

2. Add the coconut oil and cashews in the food processor and mix until the cashews turn into cashew butter. This is going to take around ten minutes and will go through several different phases. Stop every few minutes to scrape the bowl down so that everything processes completely. This will make around a cup of cashew butter.

3. Add the cashew butter to a bowl and stir in the salt, baking soda, brown rice syrup, pumpkin seeds, and almond flour.

4. Roll tablespoonfuls of the dough into balls and press them slightly to flatten. Lay them on the sheet pan and continue with the rest of the cookie dough.

5. Bake the cookies for 10 to 12 minutes, making sure that they don't burn.

6. Let the cookies cool completely before taking them off of the sheet pan. They are going to be soft and crumbly when they first come out but they will firm up as they cool.

7. Keep them in a lidded container and in the fridge so that the coconut oil doesn't melt.

Juices

The Green Machine

Serves: 1

Green apple, .5

Peeled lemon, .5

Small bunch parsley

Celery stalk

Cucumber

Dandelion greens, 2 c.

1. Juice everything and enjoy.

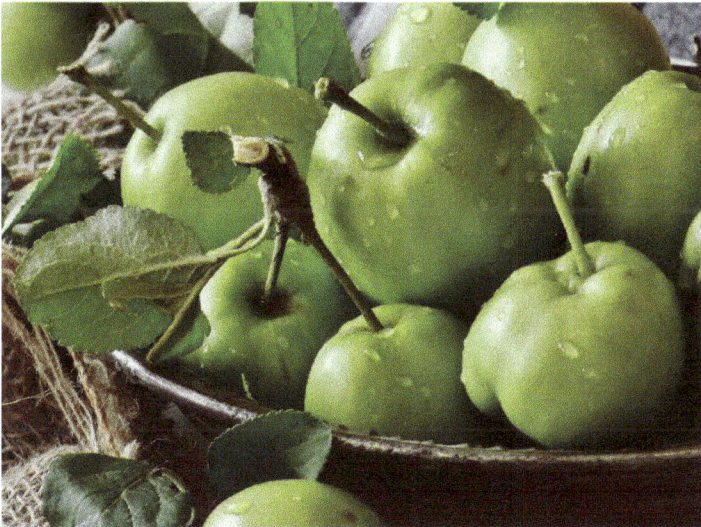

Ginger Spinach Juice

Serves: 1

Pinch sea salt

Knob of ginger

Cored green apple, .5

Peeled lemon

Scrubbed carrot

Celery stalk

English cucumber, .5

Handful baby spinach

1. Juice all of the ingredients together, stir and enjoy.

Green Juice

Serves: 1

Handful dill

Handful mint

Chunk ginger

Lime, .5

Romaine, 3 leaves

Zucchini

Celery stalk

Large cucumbers, 2

1. Juice all of the ingredients together, stir and enjoy.

Morning Energy Juice

Serves: 2

Half an apple

Red bell pepper

Ginger, .5 inch

Carrots, 2

Baby spinach, 2 c.

Melted coconut oil, 1 tbsp

Juice of a lemon

Garlic clove

Half fennel

1. Chop and wash the pepper, fennel, carrots, and greens.

2. Juice them together and then pour into a large container. Mix in the coconut oil and lemon juice. Mix and divide into two glasses.

Full Energy Juice

Serves: 2

Olive oil, 2 tbsp

Chili powder and curry powder to taste

Black pepper

Salt

Large avocado

Tomatoes, 2

Zucchini, 2

Garlic cloves, 2

Carrots, 2

Kale, 2 c.

1. Chop and wash the tomatoes, zucchini, carrots, and kale. Juice them and then juice the garlic.

2. Chop the avocado and blend the juice and avocado together in a blender and then mix in the spices.

Anti-Inflammatory Juice

Serves: 1

Red bell peppers, 2

Apple

Beets, 2

Nutmeg, .5 tsp

Cinnamon, .5 tsp

Chia seeds, two tablespoons

Oil - coconut, two tablespoons

Milk - coconut, one cup

Ginger spice, one inch

Greens of choice, 2 c.

1. Chop and wash the veggies and then juice them along with the ginger. Stir in the coconut milk, nutmeg, and cinnamon. Sprinkle with the chia seeds and enjoy.

Green Tea

Serves: 1

Juice of a lemon

Juice of 2 grapefruits

Green tea, 1 c.

1. Stir all of the ingredients together. You can add some stevia to sweeten if you would like.

Party Juice

Serves: 2

Juice of a lemon

Pear

Ginger, 1 inch

Half fennel

Broccoli florets, a few

Kale, .5 c.

Peeled cucumbers, 4

1. Clean and chop your veggies and peel the ginger and cucumber. Juice everything together and stir in the lemon juice. Divide into two glasses and enjoy.

Fat Burn Juice

Serves: 2

Cinnamon, .5 tsp

Cucumber

Beets, 2

Kale, 1 c.

Baby spinach, 1 c.

Alkaline water – if needed

1. Clean and chop your veggies and juice them together. Mix in the cinnamon. If you find that the taste is too intense, you can mix in some water to dilute it slightly. Divide into two glasses and enjoy.

Healthy Kidneys

Serves: 1

Coconut water, .5 c.

Cucumber

Kale, 1 c.

Red bell pepper

Ginger root, .5 inch

Turmeric root, .5 inch

1. Clean and chop up the ingredients and juice them together. Stir in the coconut water and enjoy.

Liver Lover

Serves: 2

Pinch salt

Ginger, 1 inch

Garlic clove

Pressed flax oil, 2 tbsp

Alkaline water, .5 c.

Parsley, .5 c.

Juice of 2 lemons

Juice of 2 grapefruits

1. Blend everything together and stir in the salt and oil. Divide into two glasses and enjoy.

Mind and Body Juice

Serves: 1

Olive oil, 1 tbsp

Fennel, .5

Turmeric, .5 inch

Ginger, .5 inch

Broccoli florets, a few

Cucumbers, 2

Celery, 2 stalks

Swiss chard, .5 c.

Kale, .5 c.

1. Wash all of the veggies and chop. Juice everything together and stir in the oil. Drink and enjoy.

Maca Juice

Serves: 2

Olive oil, 1 tbsp

Maca powder, .5 tsp

Juice of a lemon

Parsley, .5 c.

Ginger, .5 inch

Fennel slices

Tomatoes, 3

Watercress, .5 c.

1. Clean and chop your veggies and then juice them together. Put to a crystal ware then blend in with the lemon juice, oil, then maca powder. Divide into two glasses and enjoy.

Metabolism Booster

Serves: 1

Chia seeds, 1 tbsp

Mint leaves, .25 c.

Ginger, .5 inch

Cinnamon, .5 tsp

Beet

Celery, 2 stalks

Small carrot

Juice of a grapefruit

Spinach, 1 c.

1. Clean all of the ingredients and chop the carrot, spinach, beet, and celery. Juice everything together. Stir in the grapefruit juice and top with the chia seeds.

Purple Juice

Serves: 1

Pinch salt

Olive oil, 1 tsp

Juice of a lime

Juice of a lemon

Beet

Mint, .25 c.

Parsley, .25 c.

Medium cucumbers, 2

Celery, 2 stalks

1. Clean and chop the ingredients. Juice everything together and then stir in the salt, oil, lime, and lemon juice. Enjoy.

Smoothies

Kale and Avocado Smoothie

Serves: 2

Hemp seeds, 1 tbsp

Roughly chopped banana, .5

Roughly chopped avocado, .5

Stemmed kale stalks, 2

Almond milk, 1.5 c.

1. Simply place the ingredients to your blender and mix until smooth. Divide the smoothie into two glasses and enjoy.

Triple Berry Protein

Serves: 1

Pumpkin protein powder, 3 tsp

Blackberries, .33 c.

Blueberries, .33 c.

Raspberries, .33 c.

Coconut milk, 1.5 c.

1. Simply put each of the contents of the smoothie to your liquidizer then blend along till soft and nicely blended.

Pina Colada Smoothie

Serves: 1

Ice cubes, 1 c.

Pineapple chunks, 2.5 c.

Unsweetened coconut milk, .5 c.

1. Add the pineapple, coconut milk, and ice into the blender. Process until smooth and creamy.

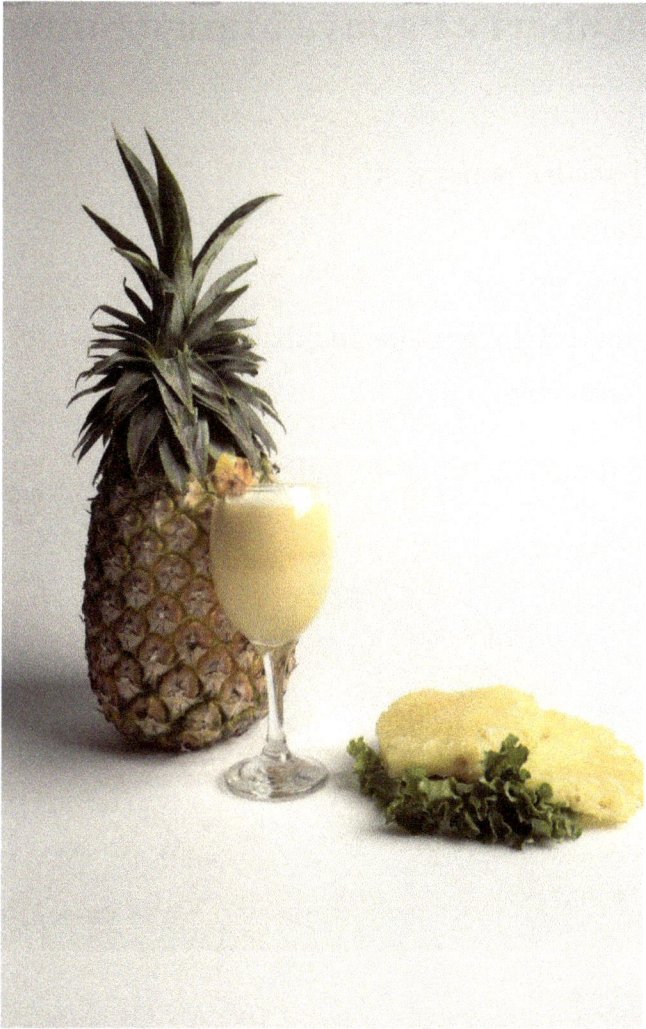

Raspberry Papaya Mango Smoothie

Serves: 1

Chopped, seeded papaya, .5

Frozen mango, .75 c.

Raspberries, .25 c.

1. Put everything to the liquidizer then process till even and creamy.

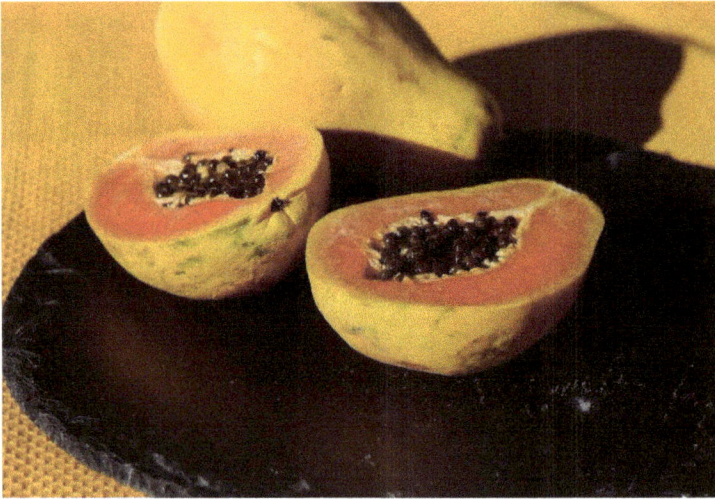

Cherry and Watermelon Smoothie

Serves: 2

Ice cubes, 5-7

Lime juice, one tablespoon

Brown rice sweetening, one tablespoon

Coconut milk, 1 c.

Dark sweet cherries, 10

Cubed watermelon, 2 c.

1. Simply add everything to your blender and mix everything together, using just enough ice to reach your desired consistency. Once smooth, pour into two glasses and enjoy.

Kiwi Hemp Seed Smoothie

Serves: 1

Ice cubes, 5-7

Hemp seeds, 2 tbsp

Blueberries, 1 c fresh or frozen

Peeled and chopped kiwi

Almond milk, 1.5 c.

1. Simply blend all of the ingredients together with enough ice to reach your desired consistency. Once everything is well combined, pour into a glass and enjoy.

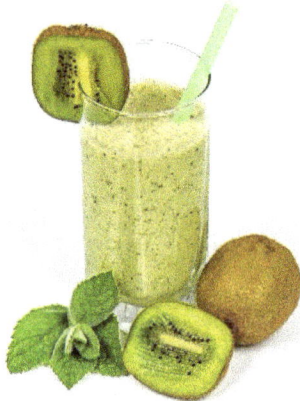

Mango Smoothie

Serves: 2

Ice cubes, 5-7

Raw cashews, .25 c.

Peeled and chopped kiwi

Chopped mango, .5 c.

Coconut milk, 1.5 c.

1. You will need a high-speed blender for this smoothie to help break up the cashews. Simply blend all of the ingredients together with enough ice to reach your desired consistency. Once well combined and smooth, pour into two glasses and serve.

Kick Start Your Diet

Starting the alkaline diet is a lot easier said than done. This section gives you ideas on how to make this new lifestyle easy to begin and stick with. Try to remember these simple principles:

- Take it slow, take baby steps, take it day by day instead of going full throttle the first day.

- Nobody is perfect. You need to enjoy life. Take a day off, enjoy your favorite treats and foods and get out there and socialize.

- You don't have to change your personality to be healthy.

This alkaline lifestyle is meant to fit into your life, not the other way around.

Five Simple Steps

- Hydration

Research shows that 90 percent of people are dehydrated and don't even know it. This has the possibility of creating a big influence on your standard of living. Many people don't like to drink water and this is probably the reason they don't feel well most of the time.

Being hydrated makes a huge difference to your immunity, vitality, energy, and health. Everything gets influenced by the quality and quantity of the water they drink. Try to filter your water until it has a pH between 8 and 9.5.

Steps to keep you hydrated:

1. Drink herbal teas like nettle and peppermint.

2. Drink lemon water: Take two cups of filtered, lukewarm water, and juice from one-fourth of a lemon. This will help cleanse your digestive system, buffer excess acids, and ignite your metabolism. As we learned before lemons are acidic in their natural state but once it gets into your system it becomes alkaline.

3. Try to drink between 6 and 18 cups of water daily. Consider your weight then split it in ½. With this range, consume those several ounces of water every day.

- Eat Green

The alkaline is all about alkaline foods. There is some conflicting information about what foods are alkaline and acid. If you stick to the lists that were given above and the 80/20 rule, you shouldn't have any problems figuring out what you should and shouldn't eat.

- Transition

Go slowly. Just about everybody out there who tries a new diet will go 100 percent out from day one but will fail within one week and it usually only takes one day.

This alkaline lifestyle isn't restrictive, isn't difficult, and is fairly simple when you have gotten your body used to it. If you try to be perfect from the beginning, you won't be able to experiment, learn, and figure out meals that work for you and your family. You might end up feeling restricted, fed up, and hungry.

It is better to transition slowly by sticking with it for a long time instead of being perfect for a couple of days and then crashing.

- Oxygen

If you can learn to do simple breathing exercises a couple times each day, you are giving your body a big hand in removing excess acids from your body. It also lets you relax, visualize, focus your mind, and just stop for the moment. Just find a place where you can sit comfortably, close your eyes, and follow this breathing exercise:

1. Inhale like this: 1, 2 (every two counts)

2. Hold onto your air for 8 counts.

3. Exhale for 4 counts.

4. Go through this exercise ten times.

- Supplements

This is the part of the alkaline diet that confuses most people. There are many supplements out there, and they all promise various things. Each one claims it is better than the next one. Here are some supplements that are recommended:

1. Omega Oils

Taking an omega-3 supplement or an oil blend that includes omega-9, 6, and 3 would be very beneficial.

2. Alkaline minerals

The best way our bodies can buffer acids is by alkaline minerals like calcium, potassium, magnesium, and sodium.

3. Alkaline water

You can create alkaline water in several different ways: adding lemon juice to your water, using pH drops, or a water ionizer.

4. Green powder

This is a combination of sprouts, vegetables, fruits, and powdered grasses while focusing on barley grass and wheat grass.

This diet is simple if you take it slow. Aim for 80/20 instead of trying to be perfect. If you allow yourself to have fun and have treats, it will make the transition smoother. Enjoy your life, have fun, and take it easy.

Keep things simple and if you make a mistake, don't beat yourself up. Take a walk, get focused, and start over. You have the rest of your life so make it interesting. Enjoy it with vitality, energy, and health that this new alkaline lifestyle will bring.

Living the Alkaline Life

Your significant other offers you a bowl of their fettuccine Alfredo. Your friend hands you a plate with a huge slice of apple pie with a scoop of ice cream on top. Your boss sends you to a conference out of town. It is hard to stick with a healthy eating plan with the people around you aren't eating healthy or if you find yourself in a situation where you might not have control of what you eat. Don't let this stress you out. Here are some tips that can help you remain on track without making others feel bad and will help you get around other food situations that might be a bit challenging.

- Happy hour

Alcoholic drinks are calorie bombs and are very acidic on the body. You need to know your options and make wise choices. If you need something bubbly, pick seltzer water which is just water with bubbles added. What's more is it is zero calories. Tonic water has 120 calories that come from nothing but sugar. When your friends want to go out, be the designated driver, your friends will thank you and won't question your choices.

- Work celebrations

Having food in the workplace is inevitable. Instead of stressing about it or letting it derail you, figure out in advance how you are going to deal with any temptations that might pop up. The best strategy is to find a support group of coworkers who are also trying to eat clean. With everyone together, you can all politely decline or bring healthier alternatives like a vegetable and fruit platter. Keep healthy snacks at your desk or in the office refrigerator so you will have something healthy when other people try to indulge. Some examples are sliced vegetables, hummus, vegetable soups, apples, whole almonds, almond butter to dip celery sticks in, and kale chips.

- Dealing with hunger

Letting yourself get hungry is the fastest way to get off track with the alkaline lifestyle. Establish an eating plan with snacks and meals. Some people need their snacks and some like to snack after every meal. You should allow natural hunger to be your guide, stress can sometimes override your natural cues but they lead us to ignore the need for nourishment. Take one day every week to get your snacks and meals planned out. This will keep your body fueled all day.

- Business dinners or lunches

You have to make your own choices and it doesn't matter what your coworkers are doing. You have free will to choose what you want to drink and eat. Every restaurant will have salads and vegetables on their menu. Many are willing to accommodate special diets. If they have a vegetable soup on the menu, order that plus add a salad or vegetables to make protein the side dish instead of the main meal. Most people don't like to appear as "high maintenance" where they work. You can make healthy boundaries for yourself and have control over what you eat. Remember the 80/20 rule if your choices aren't as ideal as they could be.

- Weekends

Having structured routines for the week helps you stick to an eating plan. When weekends roll around it can throw a wrench into the plans. There is room for splurges but remember your health goals when making choices. Stay consistent and focused. Try to continue with exercising and regular meals. You can splurge every now and then but remember portion sizes. Begin each day with a healthy breakfast, stick to the basics, and keep things simple like including vegetables, fruits, healthy fats, and lean proteins that will help you feel fuller for longer.

- Traveling

When you are away from home, sticking to a diet can be hard. You can do it if you are proactive. Take some time to research supermarkets and restaurants before you go. Pack some healthy snacks that won't spoil like apples and almonds. If you are traveling in a car, pack a cooler with tubers, avocados, seeds, fruits, and vegetables. If you will be staying at a hotel, call and request a microwave and refrigerator if they don't come with the room. You can stick to your alkaline lifestyle; all you need to do is commit, plan, and research.

- Sabotage

If your significant other doesn't approve of your new lifestyle, they might feel threatened and this causes a negative reaction. To stop this from happening, ask for their support before you begin the alkaline diet. Let them know you are living a healthier life and would like to have their support. Tell them that helping you prepare healthy meals is a great way for them to show their love. Ask them to help you find recipes and let them help plan the menu.

- Holidays

Holidays are rough on our waistlines even if you are trying to follow a special eating plan. The best thing to do is be proactive and prepare dishes that are alkaline-friendly to share at your gatherings. Remember, it is okay to eat some treats, just remember portion sizes and fill your plate with more vegetables and healthier foods.

A Few More Tips

By this point, you should have a good idea of what an alkaline diet is and how to get started. As with any diet, though, it can be difficult to really get into it and not allow yourself to fall back into old habits. To make sure you kick start your diet the best way possible, here are just a few more tips that can help to make the transition a little easier.

1. Fall in love with healthy foods

Instead of getting rid of all the foods that you love right off the bat, start to slowly add in healthy foods that will help to boost your energy and mood, like kiwi, grapefruit, berries, and green veggies. Place a chart on your fridge that shows you ten servings of good foods. Each time you eat one of the healthy foods, write it down. This will help to lower your cravings for refined sweets.

2. Fight off your cravings with healthy snacks

When you experience a craving, eat some fiber or something that is sour. This lowers your glycemic index and controls your craving. Try to keep healthy snacks on head like fruits to stay away from acidic foods like sugar and flour.

3. Start off your day with a meal that is heavy in protein to fight off sugar cravings

Instead of making dinner your biggest meal of the day, make breakfast your biggest meal. People in Japan are historically healthy, and they begin their day with fish and veggies. If you like carbs, have them first thing during the day or right have you workout. Doing this will help to keep your full and alert until your next meal without experiencing cravings. In order to figure out what your daily protein needs are, take you weight in kilograms and multiply by 0.8. A woman who weighs 135 pounds would do 62 kg x 0.8 and would need 50 grams of protein.

4. Keep a steady blood sugar level by eating every two to three hours

Make sure you keep healthy snacks on hand everywhere you go. If you make sure you have all the right stuff hidden in places like your glove compartment, purse, and office drawers, you will be less tempted to make a trip to the corner store or vending machine.

5. A crock pot will save you time and hassle during the winter

Soup makes you feel happy and warm and you can fill it with as many alkaline forming veggies as you want. Add in some good for you beans and you will get a good protein boost. Pick broth over a cream-based soup.

6. Start with green smoothies

If you begin your day with an energizing green smoothie, you will start it off with two to three servings of veggies. A lot of people struggle to eat first thing in the morning, which is when it is the most important. An alkaline smoothie will help to get your motor running and will boost your energy.

If you make sure that you follow the tips in this chapter, you will be well on your way to forming healthy habits and an alkaline diet.

Conclusion

Thank for making it through to the end of *Alkaline Diet*, let's hope it was informative and able to provide you with all of the tools you need to achieve your goals whatever they may be.

With the information that you have, you can now start a successful alkaline diet. Your body works better when it isn't acidic. The alkaline diet ensures that your body works its best. The great thing is, all of the food you can eat is tasty. With the recipes in this book, you won't have to worry about what you are going to fix for dinner. Don't wait any longer. Get started today and see your body change for the better.